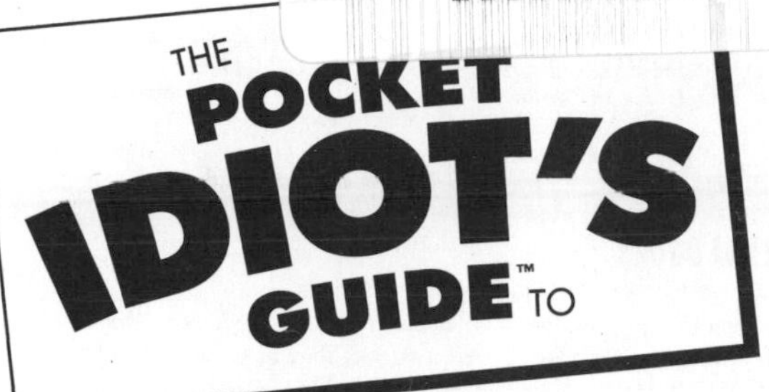

108 Yoga Poses

by Ami Jayaprada Hirschstein, RYT
Illustrated by Hrana Janto

ALPHA
A member of Penguin Group (USA) Inc.

My gratitude to all my teachers and the teachers before them: Sri Mata Amritanandamayi Devi, who showers me with Grace; John Friend, founder of Anusara Yoga; my parents, Susan and Jerry, the best role models; my husband, Ben, for his loving support and laughter; all my students, who teach me every day.—Ami

Dedicated to my mother, Phyllis Janto. Thank you for teaching me yoga as a child and suggesting I keep on doing it!—Hrana

ALPHA BOOKS

Published by the Penguin Group

Penguin Group (USA) Inc., 375 Hudson Street, New York, New York 10014, U.S.A.

Penguin Group (Canada), 10 Alcorn Avenue, Toronto, Ontario, Canada M4V 3B2 (a division of Pearson Penguin Canada Inc.)

Penguin Books Ltd, 80 Strand, London WC2R 0RL, England

Penguin Ireland, 25 St Stephen's Green, Dublin 2, Ireland (a division of Penguin Books Ltd)

Penguin Group (Australia), 250 Camberwell Road, Camberwell, Victoria 3124, Australia (a division of Pearson Australia Group Pty Ltd)

Penguin Books India Pvt Ltd, 11 Community Centre, Panchsheel Park, New Delhi—110 017, India

Penguin Group (NZ), cnr Airborne and Rosedale Roads, Albany, Auckland 1310, New Zealand (a division of Pearson New Zealand Ltd)

Penguin Books (South Africa) (Pty) Ltd, 24 Sturdee Avenue, Rosebank, Johannesburg 2196, South Africa

Penguin Books Ltd, Registered Offices: 80 Strand, London WC2R 0RL, England

International Standard Book Number: 1-59257-493-9
Library of Congress Catalog Card Number: 2005937487

08 07 06 8 7 6 5 4 3 2 1

Interpretation of the printing code: The rightmost number of the first series of numbers is the year of the book's printing; the rightmost number of the second series of numbers is the number of the book's printing. For example, a printing code of 06-1 shows that the first printing occurred in 2006.

Printed in the United States of America

Contents

Appendixes

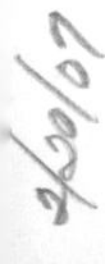

Introduction

As you practice yoga, you become part of an evolving tradition that is thousands of years old. You tap into your inherent joy, strength, and stability while bringing balance to your body and mind. You learn how to relax and become a more focused, integrated person. Yoga is a science and an art form; it is an ancient practice that is a gift from those who walked before you.

Over my years of teaching, many students have asked me if I could recommend a simple book outlining basic yoga postures generally done in classes so they can remember for the times they're practicing on their own. *The Pocket Idiot's Guide to 108 Yoga Poses* is just that—an easy reference you can take with you. Whether you're new to yoga or well practiced, you can use this guide as a supplement while you're traveling, as a work break, or to get ideas for your home practice.

Before you start, though, remember: as with any physical practice, it's important to check with your physician before embarking on any new form of exercise.

It's ideal to study with an experienced and certified yoga teacher. (For a guide, see Appendix B.) A teacher can help you work on better alignment within each pose, and he or she should be able to help you modify postures to accommodate any injuries or limitations or a pregnancy. Committing to a regular class also helps you create community, deepen your practice, be more playful, and achieve better discipline. Yoga is a path that requires tremendous discipline.

As much as it is important to go to classes for the guidance of a teacher, it is invaluable to practice regularly at home. You can move at your own pace, really cultivating your inner teacher. By exploring and playing on your own, you can find what feeds you in this moment. You can learn how to play with the edge, a fine line between honoring yourself both physically and emotionally and challenging your self-imposed limitations. How you show up in your practice on the mat reflects how you live your life.

In our society, many people feel disconnected from themselves, nature, and their community. They end up questioning themselves, their lives, jobs, and relationships. The practice of yoga is a path guiding you home. It's an amazing tool of self-exploration and expression. Yoga connects you to your essence. While you physically open and strengthen your body, you open to an understanding of your Self and the world you live in. You playfully explore your needs, strength, fears, joy, boundaries, and your tendencies of thought and action. What develops is a greater capacity for understanding and a commitment to both honoring and nourishing yourself. As you deepen this relationship with your Self, you create integration and wholeness. As you release stress and chronic tension held in the body you develop a greater capacity to enjoy the gift of life, feeling more energy to do the things you love and more joy. Vibrant and whole, you are able to creatively contribute more and enhance the world.

In both yoga and Hinduism, 108 is considered an auspicious number. The number is symbolic of the yogic journey of the integration of the Self into wholeness. In India, there are 108 shepherdesses devoted to Lord Krishna, 108 holy places of the Vaishnavas, and 108 beads on the Hindu and Buddhist rosary.

How to Use This Book

This book is divided into three basic sections:

Chapter 1 is an introduction to yoga, including its history, information on breathing, tips on alignment, and more.

Chapters 2 through 12 are broken into groups of different postures. Each of these chapters gives you illustrations and brief descriptions of the 108 poses. It's important to note, however, that each pose is only shown on one side. Be sure to repeat it on the opposite side in your practice.

Chapter 13 instructs you in four sequences, or groups of poses you can put together for a complete practice. The entire book can also be used as a longer sequence.

Throughout the book you'll see special sidebars to draw your attention. Look for these boxes to aid you in your exploration of yoga:

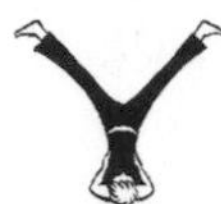

Yoga Speak

Here you'll find definitions of Sanskrit words, the language used in the ancient text of India, where yoga was born. You also find definitions for alignment, physical, and yogic terms.

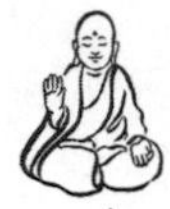

Be Mindful

Check these boxes for precautions and hints to help you avoid injury.

Acknowledgments

Thanks, Hrana, for getting me involved in this project. It was great to play with you! My gratitude to John Friend for his teachings, encouraging me to write, and graciously offering to edit my manuscript. Thanks to Gerry Simpson for her grammatical expertise. Ken Landauer, thank you so much for squeezing modeling into your busy schedule. Thanks to Barbara Boris for Iyengar classes. Thanks to Jacky Sach, Tom Stevens, Christy Wagner, and all the other editors at Alpha. Ben, I couldn't have done this without you. Thanks so much for all your support. I love you. My gratitude to Amma for guiding me to remember.—Ami

Thank you, Ami, for embarking on this journey and for modeling. It was fun to work with you! Thanks to Ken for making the time to model during a crazy busy time. Infinite thanks to my beloved Dave—for emotional and technical support, as well as eternal ingenuity. Thanks to Jacky Sach, Indra Sena, and Scott Anderson.—Hrana

Trademarks

Chapter 1

Taking the First Step: Hatha Yoga

Embarking on the practice of yoga is similar to a baby taking his or her first steps. You begin the journey inside yourself, discovering the magic of your breath, body, and spirit. Yoga gives you the tools for this exploration of the Self. As you begin to experience the gifts inherent inside you, you cultivate a deep sense of appreciation. In yoga, no one is considered an idiot. In fact, the desire to learn is cause for celebration because you are taking a step toward the truth.

The word *yoga* comes from the Sanskrit word *yuj*, which means "yoke" or "union." This signifies the union of the Self with your true nature, as well as the union of the individual with the Divine.

When you find this wholeness, you see that all creation is intertwined. The energy that pulsates within you is the Divine that flows through all living things. Just as your heart beats in your chest, *Shakti* is the life energy that makes the whole universe throb with the same beat. As you awaken to the wonders that surround you, they feed and inspire you. In response, you contribute your unique creativity, which enhances the beauty of the world. Think of the Divine as the ocean: we are all the waves, each cresting in a different way, yet each part of the whole.

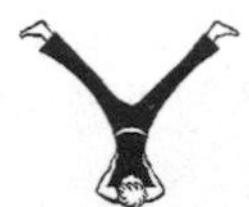

Yoga Speak

Shakti is the power and force of the Universe. It is the energy that flows through all things. Shakti is another name for the Divine.

The word *hatha* is a compound word consisting of *ha*, or "sun," and *tha*, or "moon." The word represents the joining of the opposites, the pulsation of life. You need darkness to be able to appreciate light. Without this contrast, you wouldn't see the need to make a change. All the physical exercises, regardless of their type or lineage, fall into the category of *Hatha Yoga*.

There are four types of practices or paths you can take to feel integrated within yourself and connected with the Divine. Hatha Yoga is part of the practice of *Royal*, or *Raja Yoga*. Hatha Yoga refers to all physical forms of yoga. Raja Yoga contains the Eight Limbs of Yoga (Astanga Yoga): Yama (ethical practices), Niyama (personal disciplines), Asana (physical postures), Pranayama (breathing exercises), Pratyahara (withdrawal of external sensory input), Dharana (concentration), Dhyana (meditation), and Samadhi (oneness with the Divine). *Jnana Yoga* is knowledge yoga, the study of sacred text; *Bhakti Yoga* is the yoga of devotion; and *Karma Yoga* is the yoga of action.

The Roots of Yoga

The practice of yoga is an ancient one. Yoga's roots can be traced back to texts as old as 3000 B.C.E. Mostly an oral tradition handed down from teacher to student, surviving texts on Hatha Yoga were not written until much later. Historians do not agree on yoga's exact age. One of the most famous text that codified about yogic philosophy, Patanjali's *Yoga Sutras*, was written in approximately 200 C.E. The first text written about the physical practice, the *Hatha Yoga Pradipika* by Svatmarama, was not written until around the fourteenth century. Since then, the practice of yoga has been evolving and unfolding.

Over the centuries, many schools of yogic philosophy and lineages of Hatha Yoga have developed. (Think of Hatha Yoga as a tree with many limbs and branches.) Each school views the journey of yoga in a different way. Each believes that the path of yoga is a path to experiencing our fullness (hence the word *union*). You are complete and you are whole; you have just forgotten this. Yoga is a journey of remembrance and Truth.

When you're in physical pain, you have little energy to contribute to yourself, your job, your family, or your community. When you feel well, you can put time and energy into being a better person and contributing more to those around you.

Through Hatha Yoga, you learn how to have better posture; deeper breath; and increased circulation, strength, and stamina. You feel physically better, aligning with the intention to be a stronger, more radiant and joyful being.

Are you ready to take that first step?

Finding a Teacher for You

As mentioned in the introduction, it is important to study with a certified teacher in addition to developing your own practice. The many different Hatha Yoga styles evolved out of the different lineages of teachers. This variety of styles emerged out of the need for different personality types to have practices that created balance for them. Some practices are so diverse that they barely resemble each other. If this isn't confusing enough, each teacher has his or her own unique approach to the style he or she teaches.

With all this variety, how do you find a class that works for you? Explore! My journey through yoga has taken me through four different styles until I found the style that worked for me. As I changed, my needs shifted and it was essential for my practice to change as well. It took me years of taking classes with a wide variety of teachers to find teachers that really spoke to me. This book is influenced by those teachers who have made me the teacher I am today. This book especially reflects my training with John Friend in Anusara Yoga, which combines therapeutic alignment with heart-centered instruction. So shop around; experiment with different teachers and styles until you find what's right for you.

In Appendix B, I give you a list of resources for finding certified teachers in your area.

Breathing: A Partnership

Breathing is the foundation for any yoga practice. The Sanskrit word for "breath" is *Prana*, which also means "life force energy." You receive Prana from things that enhance the flow of your vitality: breath, sunlight, water, food, as well as things that inspire and feed your soul and creativity. All things pulsate with Prana. Even the Universe has this expansion and contraction. Pause for a moment and feel your breath. Rather than forcing in the inhalation, open your lungs and heart to receive the breath. For a brief moment, feel the charge and fullness of a bright *inner body*. Keeping your body expansive, relax and allow the breath to flow out, noticing how your skin softens.

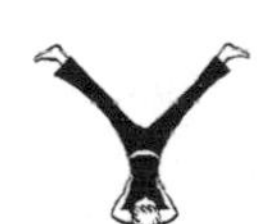

Yoga Speak

Prana is life force energy. *Prana* is also synonymous with *breath*. The **inner body** is the energetic body, which can physically swell, expanding the body to contain more prana. Your **outer body,** or skin, is like a cloth draping over your internal expansiveness. You want to relax and soften your body without losing this extra prana.

You can receive Prana from other life-charging forces such as the sun. As you inhale, know that you're breathing the same air as all living beings. Green plants provide you with oxygen, and you reciprocate with carbon dioxide. The sun that shines upon you is the same sun that brightens all living things. As you exhale, offer back out just as much as you've received. Allow your breath to connect you to the interwoven web of life. Step into the flow of life's creation.

Balancing Action

No *asana*, or posture, should ever feel painful. Pain is the body's way of letting you know that something is out of alignment. However, you may feel sore as you develop new muscular strength. Hatha Yoga teaches the art of balance. You want to open in a new way, yet you do not want to push yourself too far. This fine line is constantly shifting. Yoga can teach you how to listen to your needs in each moment. As you become more sensitive, you will understand how to both honor and shift your boundaries.

Every pose should have *balanced action*, or a balance of:

- Engaging and softening
- Integration and extension
- Receiving and giving
- Discipline and spontaneous play
- Taking it to the next level and respecting your limitations

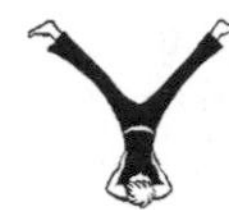

Yoga Speak

In Sanskrit, ***asana*** literally means "seat." Asanas are Hatha Yoga postures. When you have a balance of energies within an asana, you have **balanced action.**

Integration Is the Key

One of the common misconceptions about yoga is that it is entirely made up of stretching. Many people come to me saying, "I can't do yoga. I am too inflexible." Anyone can do yoga if it is modified correctly. Physiologically, it is important to engage your muscles before stretching. Then your muscles and ligaments will open together. When you only stretch, you can stretch just the ligaments, opening yourself up to injury. Unlike muscles, once ligaments are stretched, they cannot shrink back. They become like overstretched rubber bands and are weak. When you engage muscles and then stretch, the muscles help keep the ligaments from overstretching.

Aligning with the Optimal You

Some principles of alignment will help you be as you were intended to be: open, strong, graceful, creative, happy, and free. When you're out of alignment, you're partially cut off from the natural pulsation. As you align with this flow, you take a step toward being the optimal you. Each of the following Anusara alignment principles adds to the next:

1. Open to Grace It's our attitude that's most fundamental to our practice. Set an intention for your practice—perhaps you'd like to offer your practice to a friend in need, a teacher, or yourself. Maybe your practice is a celebration. For that intention, open to receive your breath, feeling your body shine from the inside out. You swell with the fullness of life. Set your foundation for this intention by being sure you're standing evenly, with your *feet parallel*. Without losing your brightness, soften into this moment.

2. Muscular Energy You align with this intention by drawing in, feeling your muscles engaging. Your muscles hug evenly to your bones; you draw from the periphery of your limbs into the core of your body. *Isometric exercises* are used to help engage your muscles. Celebrate your innate strength!

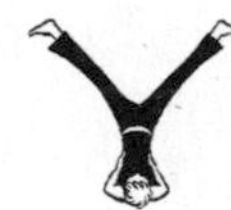

Yoga Speak

When you energetically draw parts of your body in toward each other without moving them, your muscles engage. Try hugging your legs energetically in toward each other without physically moving them. You'll feel your inner legs engage in this **isometric exercise.**

3. Inner Spiral Imagine a tornadolike spiral that begins at your feet and expands, widening up your legs, into your waist. The action turns your thighs slightly in toward each other and then back and apart so that the top of your thighs move back and the back of your pelvis widens behind you. Feel awkward? Don't worry—this expanding spiral combines with the next action to align the hips and back.

4. Outer Spiral Keeping your inner thighs back, subtly *scoop* your tailbone. You'll feel a toning of your buttocks. This spiral moves opposite of the Inner Spiral yet complements it.

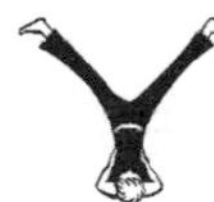

Yoga Speak

Scooping your tailbone roots your tailbone straight down. Often the tailbone sticks out behind you like a happy dog wagging its tail. This indicates an overarching of the back. Keeping the top of your thighs back, draw your tailbone subtly down so it points toward the earth.

5. Organic Energy Extend your offering, your arms a radiant expression of your heart, your legs lengthening from the core of the pelvis.

In addition to these Five Principles, the *Focal Point* is found within each pose. This point of alignment feeds the power of each pose, balancing Muscular and Organic energy. The Focal Point is where the received energy pools and collects; then it extends out from that point. Prana or Shakti is received, channeled, and offered back. There are three Focal Points, but only one is active in each pose. They are …

- The core of the pelvis.
- The bottom of the energetic heart—center of sternum.
- The center upper palate.

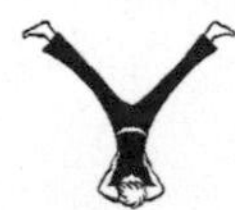

Yoga Speak

The **Focal Point** is where energy is directed, collected, and radiated out in an asana. Only one of the three Focal Points is active in each pose.

Whichever Focal Point is closest to weight bearing determines which Focal Point is active. For example, for most standing and seated poses, it's the pelvis. For hand balances and inversions, it is the heart—except in inversions where the head is the base, in which case it is the upper palate. When all three Focal Points are weight bearing equally the pelvic focal point is used.

Chapter 2

Planting the Seed: Focusing and Centering Yourself

Your breath and your intention are the most important parts of your yoga practice, and these two go hand in hand. Taking time before you move helps you settle into this moment to focus and center yourself. It's like you're planting a seed. This is the time when you set the foundation of your practice so you can enjoy the fruit of that intention that springs forth from that seed.

You want your yoga practice to be a refuge from your busy life. You want to be able to experience the riches life's gifts have to offer. It is easy to miss these or take these gifts for granted in a fast-paced life. Take a few minutes to just sit and be present to the moment instead of being active. Enjoy your breath; enjoy that you are alive. You are surrounded by abundance. Your body is a miracle—how it moves, what you are able to accomplish with it, and how all the systems in your body work together to keep you alive. How beautiful is the world of which we are an intricate part of.

Taking Your Seat

Yoga classes often begin with chanting *Om*. When you chant Om, you are acknowledging that you're part of the interwoven web of life. A living, pulsating force interconnects you with all other living things while your mind, fears, and stress separate you from yourself and this bigger picture. Think of yoga as a moving form of meditation that connects you to the web of life.

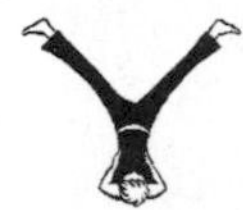

Yoga Speak

Om is the sound of the vibration of the Universe. Often chanted at the beginning and end of a yoga class, it is an acknowledgment that we are all part of the interwoven web of life.

One of Patajali's Yoga Sutras says, "*Sthira sukham asanam*—Postures should be steady and comfortable." You'll have an easier time sitting and becoming focused if you can be comfortable. Here are some tips on getting comfortable as you sit in the beginning of your yoga practice:

- If your lower back tends to round backward or if you have tight hips, you should be sitting on a pillow or folded blanket.
- If your knees are higher than your hip creases, you need to sit up higher. If this is

still uncomfortable, you can even sit in a chair.

- Try shifting your weight to one buttock and pulling the flesh of the opposite buttock away from your sitz bone so you have more contact between your bone and the floor (or blanket). Repeat on the opposite side.
- With your hands on the floor by your hips, as you inhale, press down into the earth and your spine will elongate. Keeping this length, rest your hands on your thighs and soften.
- Your shoulder blades should be flat on your back, your neck in line with your spine (we often pull our heads forward), and chin parallel to the earth. As you extend up through the crown, root your tailbone down into the earth.

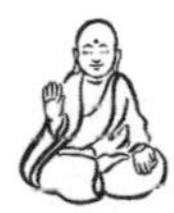

Be Mindful

Be sure your back doesn't collapse. It shouldn't be rounding backward. How do you know if your blanket or pillow is high enough? Your knees should be no higher than the creases of your hips. If they're higher, you need to sit up higher. If you have knee problems, try rolling a sock behind your knees so when you bend them, the sock creates space in the back of your knee.

Centering and Opening to Receive

Now focus on your breath, inhaling through your nose and exhaling through your nose. As you inhale, feel the breath expanding your lungs, heart, and chest. You are being nourished by Prana. As you exhale, feel the tension dropping away as your body relaxes and lets go. When your mind wanders, notice the thought and with your exhalation, let it go, coming back to the sensation of the next inhalation. Allow yourself to really settle into this breath.

Once you have become centered, choose an intention for your practice. Your intention might simply be to experience the moment. Perhaps you would like to celebrate life's fullness or offer your practice to someone who is struggling. If you are the one who is struggling, your intention could be to just be fully present to that struggle or to nourish yourself. Maybe your practice is a contemplation of why you do yoga. Whatever your intention is, it infuses your practice with meaning.

Simple Seated Pose/Sukhasana

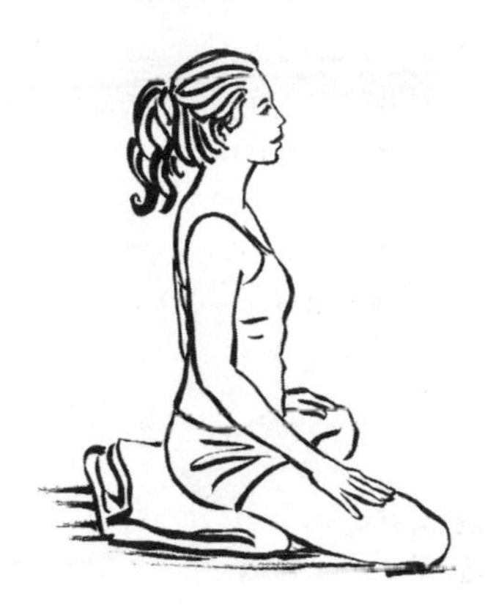

1. Sitting up on your blanket or pillow, bend your knees, crossing your legs at your ankles or shins. Your hands rest comfortably on your thighs. Focus on your breath, and allow it to fill you.
2. Hugging your legs in toward each other, gently turn your thighs in toward each other and down toward the floor. Now scoop your tailbone, and you'll feel more back support.
3. Continue drawing your tailbone down as you expand again, extending through your crown. Your sternum lifts, and your shoulders and ribs soften.
4. Focus on your breath, and create an intention for your practice.

Seated Pose Variation

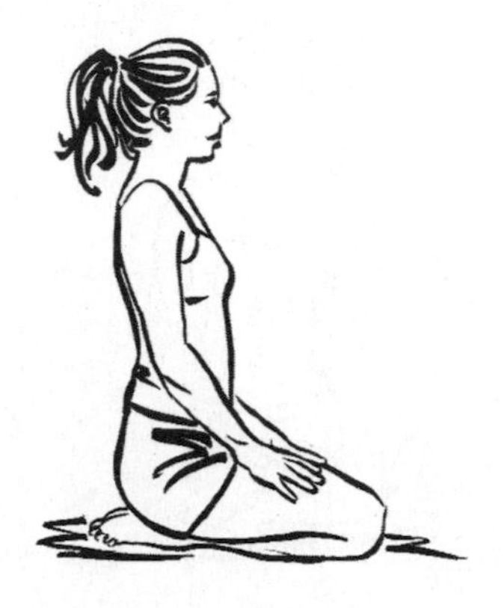

1. With your legs together, kneel on the floor. Now sit back on your heels. Your toes should be pointing straight back. Your hands rest comfortably on your thighs.
2. Sitting up tall and comfortably, deepen your breath. What are you dedicating your practice to?

Seated Pose with Full Yogic Breath

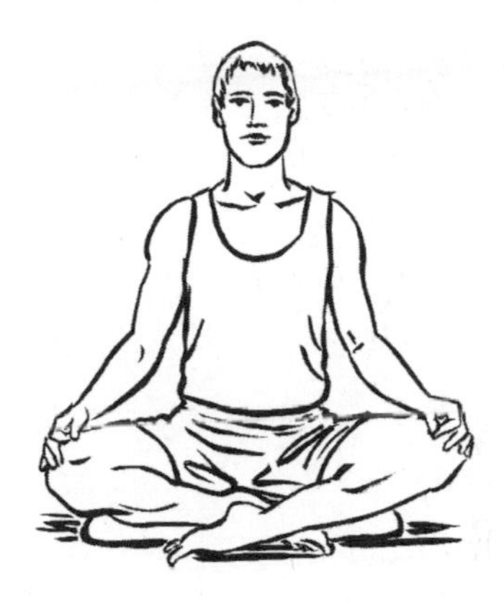

1. Take a comfortable and tall seated position.
2. As you inhale through your nose, feel your breath washing up your spine. First your diaphragm and belly fill with Prana, then the breath moves into the lower half of your lungs, and finally into your upper chest.
3. As you exhale, feel the breath washing down your body. It releases first from your upper chest, then your lower lungs, and finally your diaphragm and belly.
4. Make your inhalation and exhalation even in length. Your epiglottis, inside your throat, constricts slightly so your breath even sounds like ocean waves washing up and down the shore.

Chapter 3

Welcoming the Sun: Warm-Ups for Body and Breath

Get your body moving! Warm-ups wake up the body; increase circulation; lubricate the joints; and warm the muscles, ligaments, and connective tissue. The body becomes open and ready for practice. Injuries often occur when the body is not warmed-up properly, so be sure to include warm-ups in your yoga practice.

You also need to cater your practice to the condition of your body, time of day, and seasons. You may already notice that you tend to be stiffer in the morning and more open during the day and night. This occurs because you've been using your body all day. If you sit for long hours in a chair, you'll notice that the longer you sit still, the more achy and stiff your body becomes. As your body "cools" when you're still, in cool weather, you need to spend more time warming up. In hot weather, you become more flexible and open, so you don't need to warm up as much.

In my Gentle Yoga classes, nearly the whole class is devoted to warm-ups. This is ideal for people who are arthritic, always achy, or working with severe injuries or limitations. If your joints pop and crack, increasing warm-ups, especially circular movements, will help. I also recommend using warm-ups to wake up your body as you start the day.

Try circling your joints: ankles, knees, hips, shoulders, and wrists—but not your neck. The neck is not a ball-and-socket joint and should not be circled. Instead, you can nod your head "yes" and "no" and tilt your head from side to side. All these motions stimulate *synovial fluid*, which is the shock-absorber of all the joints. Doing this regularly helps prevent injuries. Remember to circle in both directions.

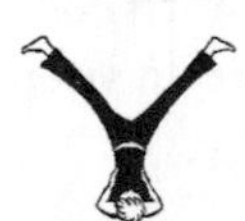

Yoga Speak

Synovial fluid is a lubricating fluid secreted by the synovial membrane. Both the membrane and the fluid protect the joints.

Sun Breaths

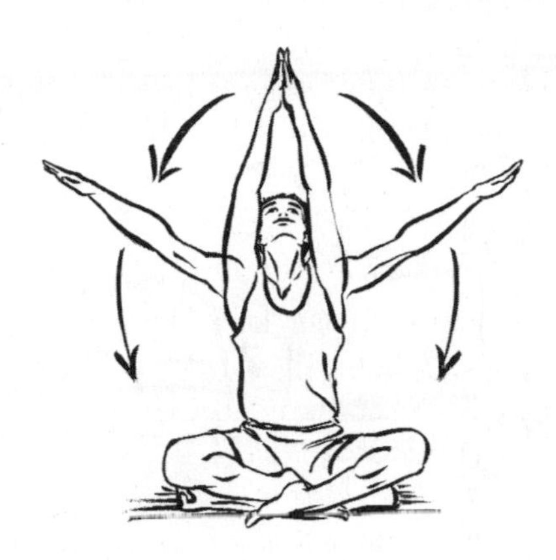

1. Sit in Simple Seated Pose/Sukhasana or stand in Mountain/Tadasana, resting your arms at your sides.
2. As you inhale, let your arms ride the wave of your breath, out to your sides, and up overhead.
3. As you exhale, release your arms with your breath.
4. Allow your movement to follow your breath for 5 to 10 breaths.

Table Position

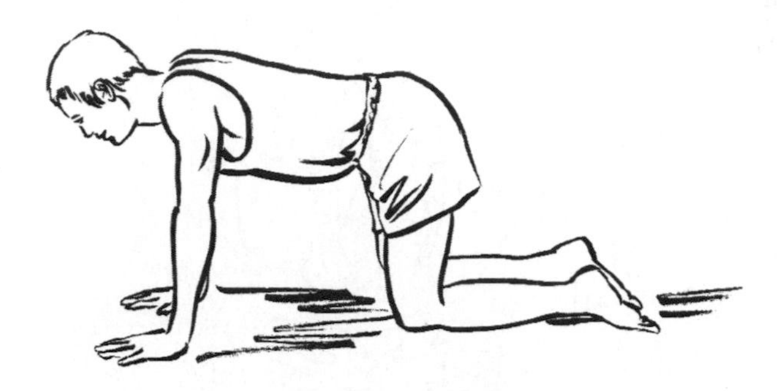

1. Come onto your hands and your knees. Place your hands on the floor shoulder-width apart and directly under your shoulders. Move your knees hip-width apart. Open to receive your breath as your body expands with Prana.
2. To contain that energy, isometrically (energetically, without physically moving) swipe your hands and knees into each other. As you draw energetically from your hands into your heart, your shoulder blades will come onto your back.
3. Keeping your arms straight and your body inflated, offer your light back out as you let your energetic heart (sternum area) soften down.

Cat

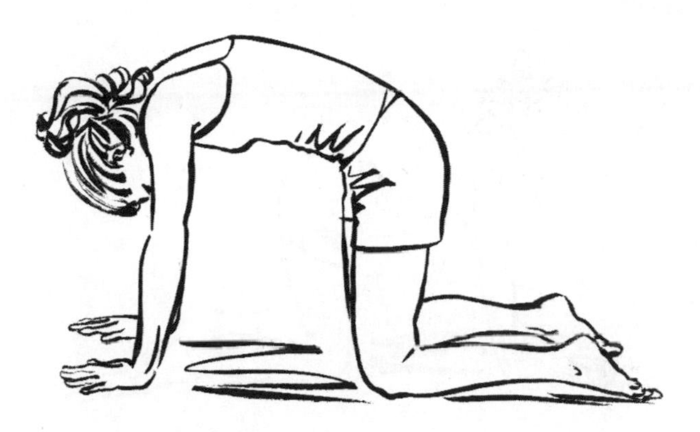

1. From Table Position, exhale as you draw your chin into your chest and round your back up to the sky.
2. This pose mimics a cat when it gets surprised. Rounding your back is not recommended if you have any herniated discs.

Cow

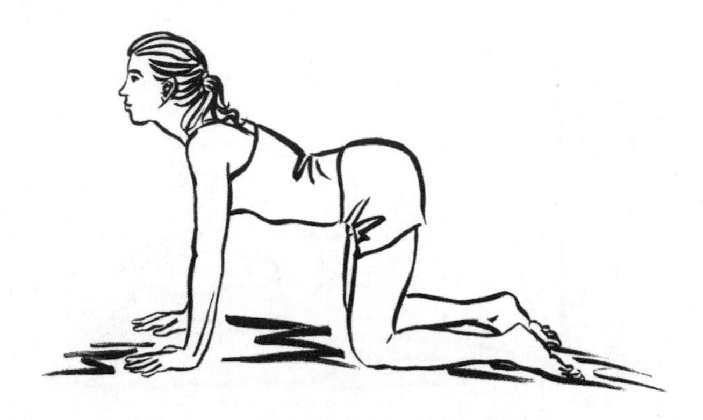

1. From Cat or Table, inhale as you press your buttocks up and look up so your back is gently arched.
2. Try flowing from Cat into Cow, inhaling in Cow and exhaling in Cat and repeating a few times as you move with your breath.

Child's Pose/Balasana

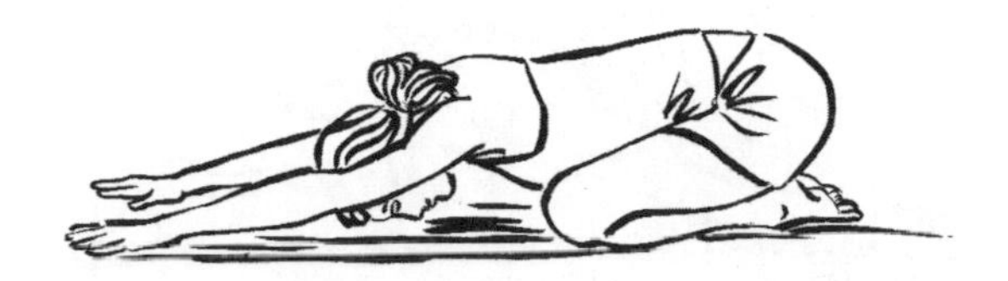

1. Begin on your hands and knees (Table Position).
2. Bring your buttocks back to your heels, and release your head onto the floor (or toward it if you can't make it all the way to the floor).
3. Your arms are over your head, along the floor. Place your fingertips on the floor.
4. First, plug into the energy that feeds all things by drawing from your fingers into your heart.
5. Keeping your shoulders in their sockets, create an offering. Stretch from your heart back out through your arms.
6. Draw your buttocks back to your heels to open your whole spine. Enjoy the freedom of your breath as you elongate your lungs. Hold for at least five breaths.

Puppy Stretch

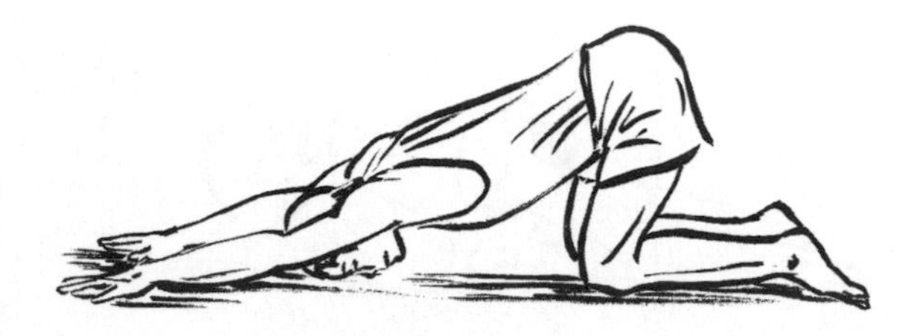

1. From Child's Pose, lift your hips in the air 1 foot higher.
2. Receive the gift of the breath and then actively draw that energy in from your fingers into your heart, charging your pose.
3. Lift your armpits away from the floor as you pull your shoulder blades onto your back.
4. As you exhale, offer back out as you melt your heart and extend from your heart out through your fingers and back through your buttocks, lengthening your whole spine. Hold for at least five breaths.

Downward Facing Dog/ Adho Mukha Svanasana

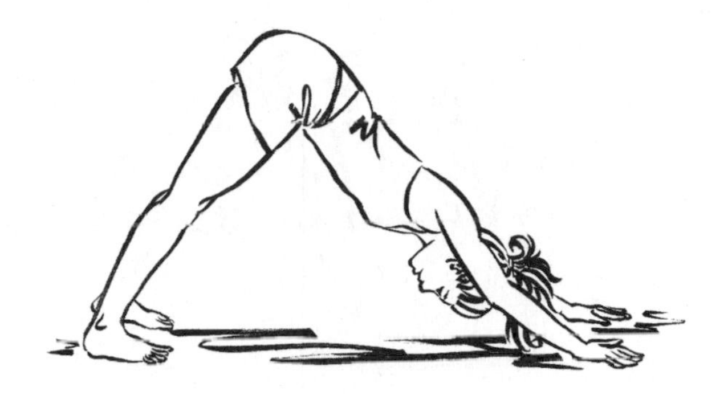

1. From Child's Pose, curl your toes under. As you inhale, receive your birthright and draw that energy from your fingers into your heart, allowing your shoulder blades to come flat onto your back as your heart is strengthened and nourished.
2. By lifting your elbows and armpits away from the floor, engaging your shoulders will be easier. Keeping your shoulders on your back, exhale and allow your energetic heart (sternum) to soften graciously.
3. Stretch your legs straight, reaching your hips up and back.
4. From your heart, offer back your strength as you extend out through your hands and elongate your whole body.
5. Extend your heels back and down. Hold for five breaths to one minute.

Forward Bend Flow/ Uttanasana Flow

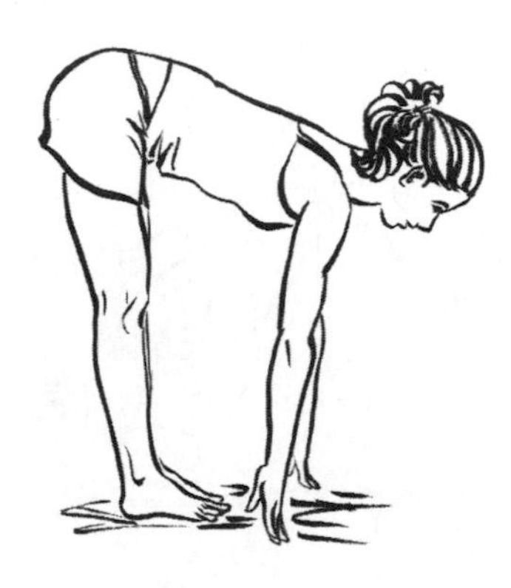

1. Stand with your feet hip-width apart and parallel. Bow forward, hinging at your hips. (If you're coming from Downward Facing Dog, just step forward.)
2. Touch the floor with your fingertips, hands on either side of your feet. If you can't touch the floor, rest your hands on your legs.
3. Inhale and open to receive your fullness, lifting to a flat back with your chest parallel to the floor. Your arms lengthen as you extend.
4. As your body swells from the inside out, extend your heart out in offering, elongating your spine.
5. Keeping this expansiveness, exhale and bow in a self-honoring fold forward.
6. Continue this a few times: inhale and lift; exhale and bow.

Full Forward Bend/Uttanasana

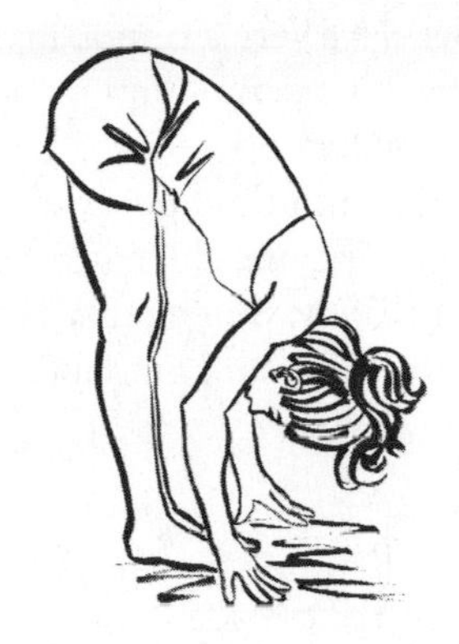

1. Stand with your feet hip-width apart and parallel. Draw your legs energetically in toward each other and up into the core of your pelvis as if you are pulling on stockings.
2. Bow forward, hinging at your hips.
3. Keeping your muscular energy in your legs, create balance by offering your energy back to the earth, lengthening your legs from your pelvis down into your feet and extending your sitz bones up as your feet root down.
4. Touch the floor with your fingertips, hands on either side of your feet, or hold onto your legs if you can't reach the floor. Hold for five breaths or more.

Sun Salutation/Surya Namaskar

Sun Salutations are a series of postures that flow into each other. This *vinyasa* has many variations and is a popular warm-up because it works each major muscle group in the body. Surya Namaskar is a great way to welcome the day, inviting sun energy into your body. Sun energy is invigorating, charging, and warming and gets the body's systems stimulated.

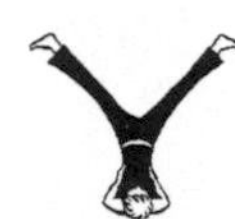

Yoga Speak

Vinyasa is a flowing form. Each pose is linked to the next so that they form a routine.

It's a good idea to do other warm-ups before Sun Salutation, as the backbends and forward bends can be too extreme to begin with.

The Sun Salutation begins and ends with the Mountain Pose/Tadasana with the hands held in *Anjali Mudra.* Tadasana is the foundation of all standing poses. Some basics things about to remember in Mountain are:

Keep your feet parallel. Line up your second toe with the middle of your ankles and middle of your knees (big toe being toe number one and pinky toe being toe number five). For some, this will result in a slightly pigeon-toed position.

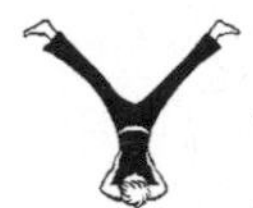

Yoga Speak

Sun Salutations begin with the hands in **Anjali Mudra,** or together in a prayer position over the heart. *Anjali* literally means "to extend forth offering."

Keep your *Four Corners of the Feet* activated. Ground the fleshy mound where your foot meets your big toe (big toe mound, not the big toe itself), the inner edge of your heel, the fleshy mound where the foot meets your pinky toe (pinky toe mound), and the outer edge of your heel on each foot. When the Four Corners of each foot are grounded, your arches, kneecaps, and thighs lift and engage. Keeping the arches lifted, relax and spread your toes.

Keep your legs both rooting down into the earth and extending up to the sky.

Mountain Pose/Tadasana

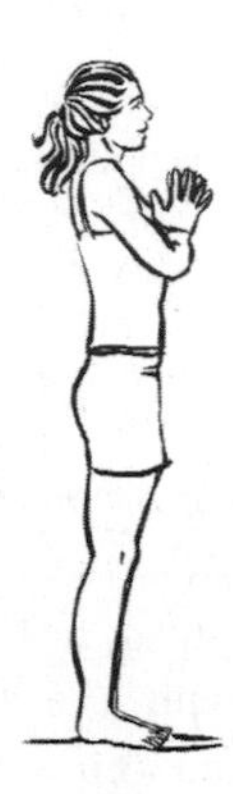

1. Stand with your feet an inch or two apart and parallel. Open to receive your inherent fullness, allowing your breath to fill your body as your chest lifts and expands. As you exhale, your outer body softens over your internal brightness.
2. Align with your innate strength; isometrically hug your legs in toward each other; and draw from your feet up into the core of your pelvis.
3. Keeping this engagement, turn your thighs slightly in toward each other and back. The top of your thighs move back and the back of your pelvis broadens in Inner Spiral.
4. Scoop your tailbone (Outer Spiral) and extend out through your legs down into the Four Corners of each foot.
5. Place your hands together over your heart in Anjali Mudra, and offer out your intention that you set for your practice.

Arch Back

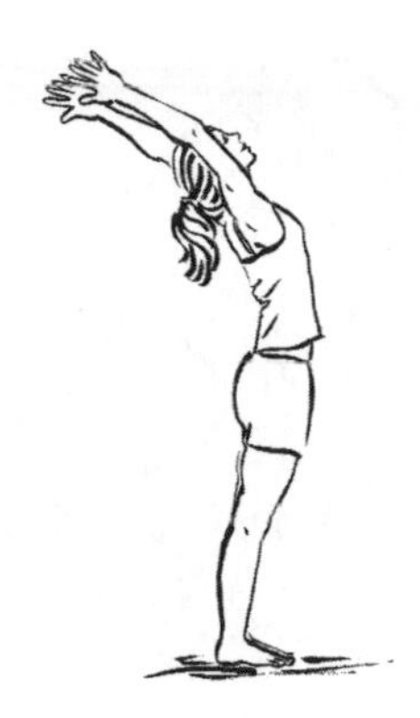

1. From Tadasana, inhale your arms up, scoop your tailbone, and offer out your heart, lifting and expanding it while arching your back.

Swan Dive Forward

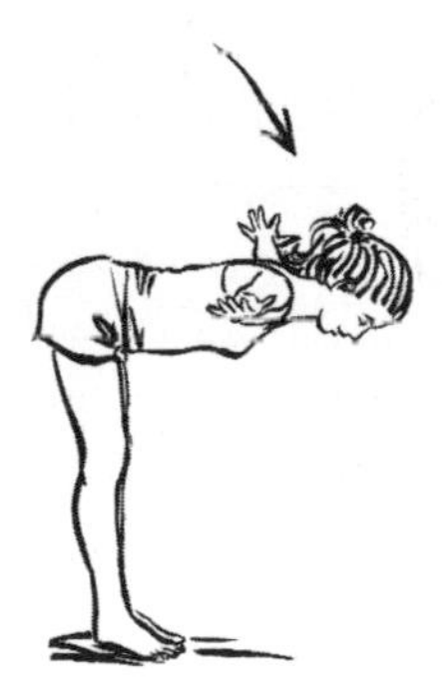

1. From Arch Back, with your exhalation, release your arms as you swan dive forward, hinging at the hips.

Forward Bend/Uttanasana

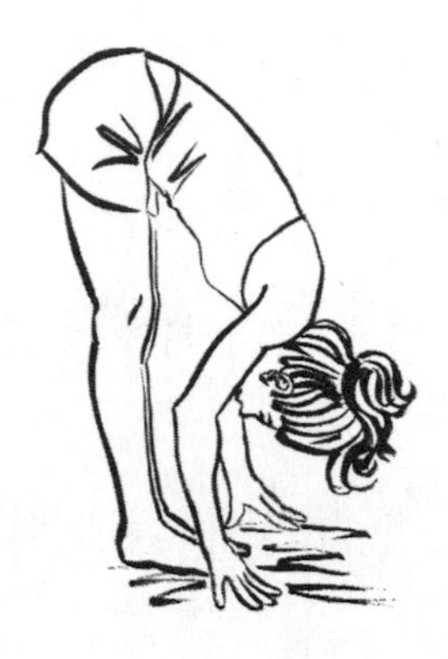

1. As you inhale, lift up halfway and, reaching out your heart's desire, lengthen your spine.
2. As you exhale, bow again in a Full Forward Bend.

Lunge—Right Leg Back

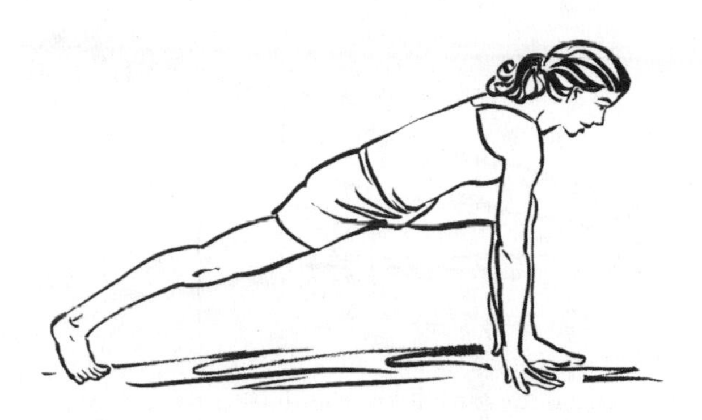

1. From Forward Bend, step your right leg back. Your left knee should be over your ankle. Your right heel should be off the floor.
2. Draw your legs in energetically to each other and into the core of your pelvis.
3. As you keep hugging your legs in, extend from your pelvis out through your right heel back toward the floor, through your right hip, which reaches forward and out through your heart, creating one line of energy.
4. Pull your left hip crease back and down to square your hips.

Plank

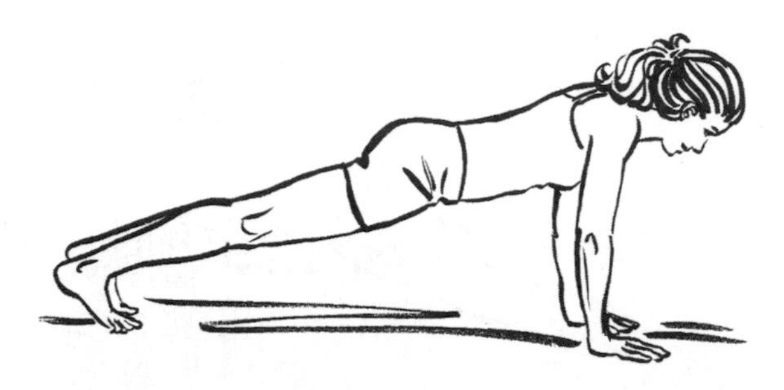

1. From Lunge, step your left leg back, bringing your body parallel to the floor. Be sure your hands are directly under your shoulders.
2. Isometrically swipe your hands and feet in toward each other.
3. Extend out through your heels and tailbone.
4. Keep your arms long as you *melt your heart.*

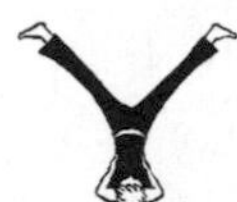

Yoga Speak

When your energetic heart softens and expands without losing shoulder alignment or losing your inner expansiveness, this is called **melting the heart.** Think of an abundant bunch of grapes weighing down a vine. You have much to be thankful for, so your heart swells with gratitude for this abundance.

Eight-Point Prostration

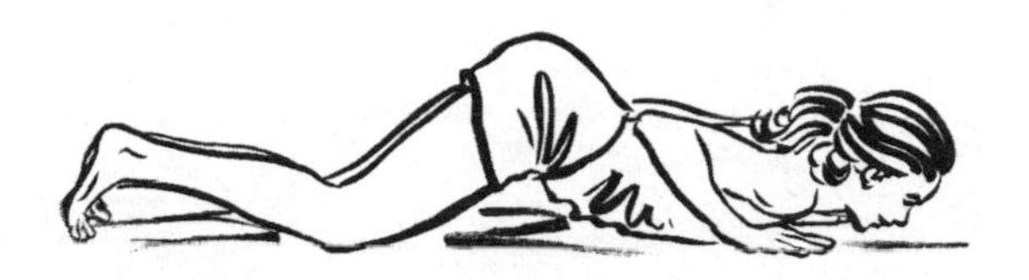

1. From Plank, drop your knees, chest, and chin to the floor.
2. Your buttocks stay pointing up into the air.

Four-Limbed Staff/Chaturanga Dandasana

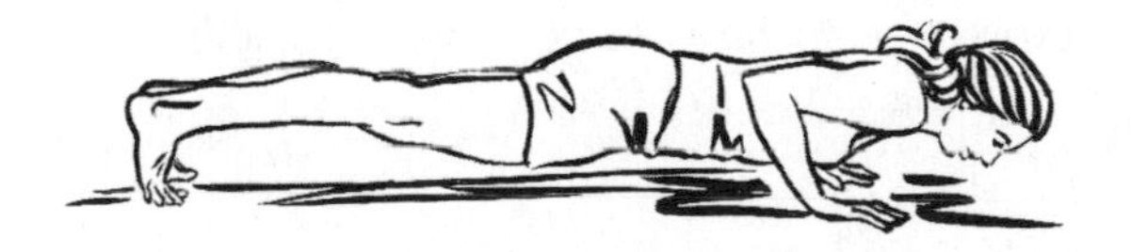

If you want more of a challenge, you can replace this pose with Eight Point Prostration..

1. From Plank, slowly lower yourself to 1 inch away from the floor.
2. Your whole body should be level. Watch that your shoulder blades are flat on your back and that you're not lifting up your buttocks.

Half Cobra/Ardha Bhujangasana

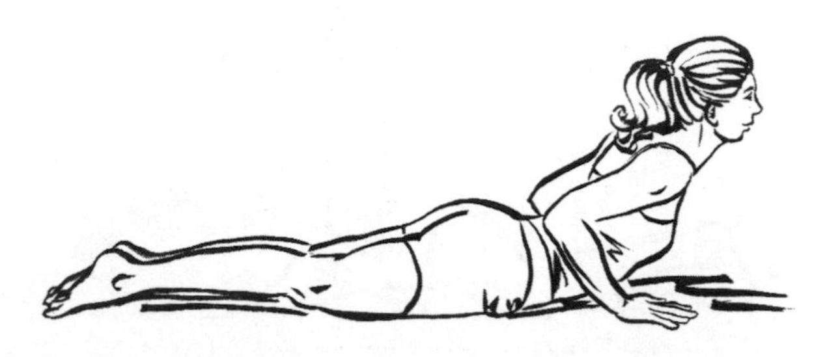

1. From Eight Point Prostration or Four Limbed Staff, drop your pelvis onto the floor. Check that your hands are still under your shoulders.
2. Lift your head and chest, extending your heart forward.
3. Hug your shins in and down, scooping your tailbone as you claw the floor, drawing your fingers in toward your heart so your heart can shine, expanding out with offering.

Cobra/Bhujangasana

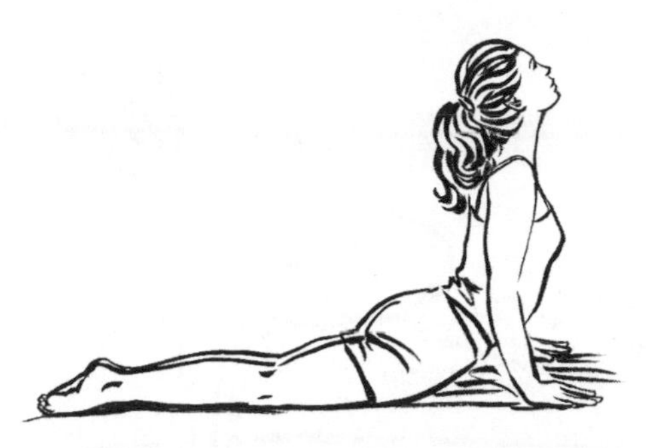

1. This is a deeper variation of Half Cobra. If you're more flexible you can lift up higher.
2. Try to bend more from the back of your heart and less from your lower back.
3. Maintain your shoulder blades flat on your back.

Downward Facing Dog/Ado Mukha Svanasana

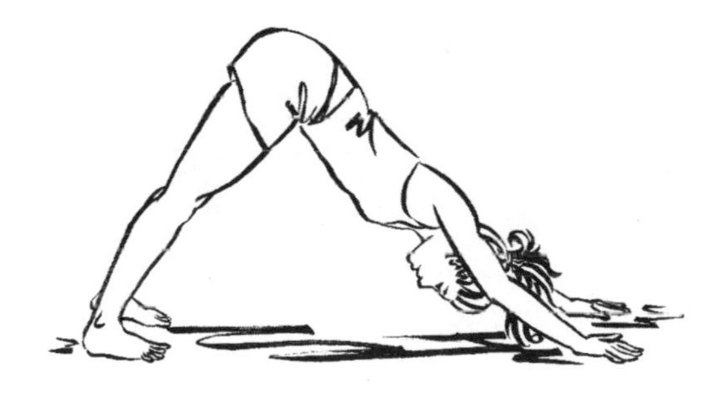

1. From Cobra, curl your toes under and reach your hips up and back, coming back into Downward Facing Dog.

Lunge—Right Leg Forward

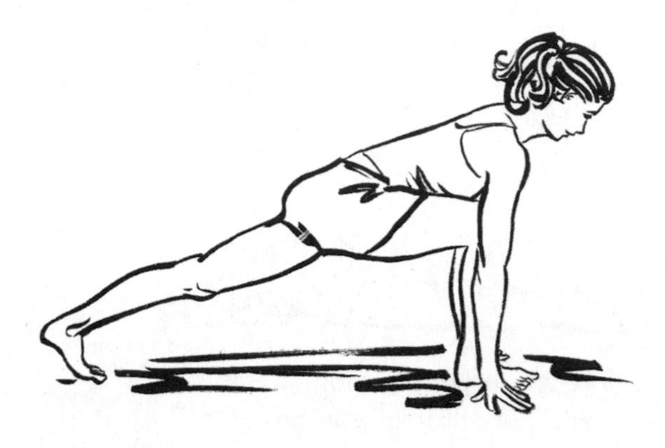

1. From Downward Facing Dog, step your right foot forward. If you can't step in between your hands, grasp your ankle and help move it forward.
2. Your right knee should be over your right ankle.

Forward Bend/Uttanasana

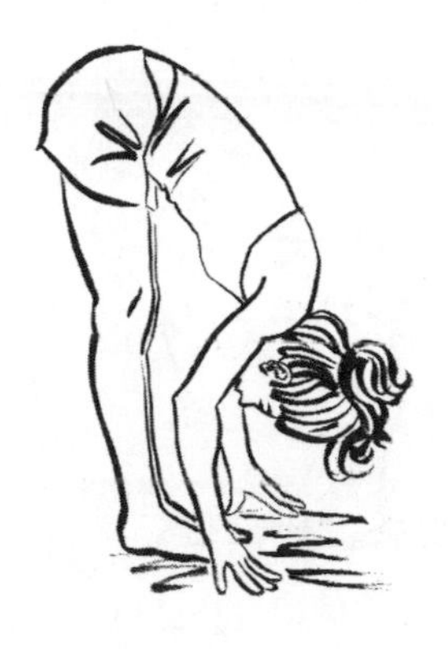

1. From Lunge, step your left foot forward so you're back in Standing Forward Bend. Be sure your feet are parallel.
2. Engage your legs fully as you inhale, receiving the gift of the breath and lifting your chest halfway.
3. Exhaling, bow gratefully with the breath.

Reverse Swan Dive

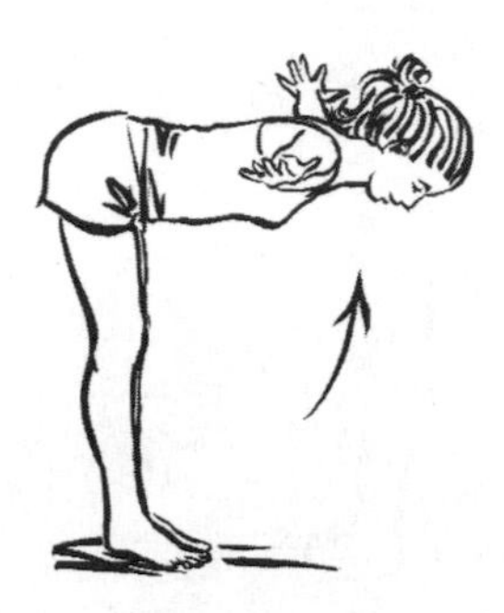

1. From Forward Bend, inhale your arms out to T position as you come up to standing with a flat back.

Arch Back

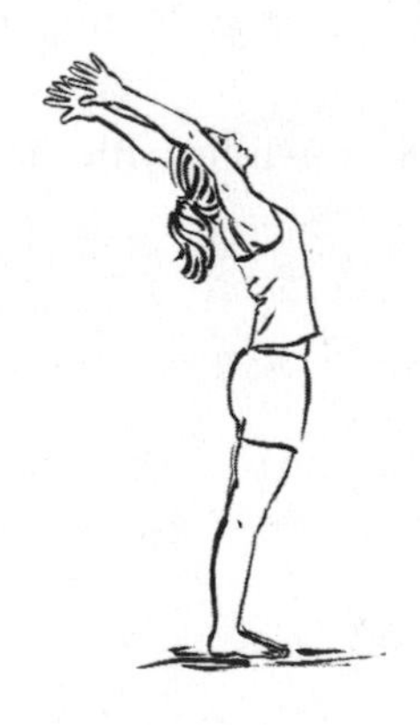

1. From Reverse Swan Dive, sweep your arms over head and arch back, opening your heart and lungs while rooting your tailbone and legs.

Mountain Pose/Tadasana

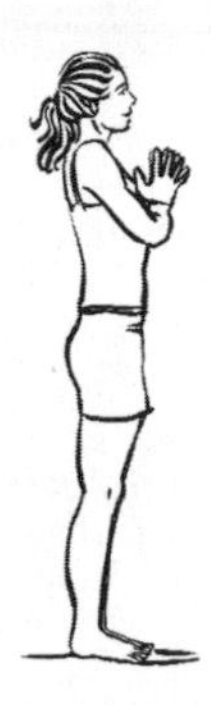

1. From Arch Back, as you exhale, release your arms and stand tall, back in Mountain Pose.

You have now done half of one Sun Salutation. Repeat on the left side, stepping your left leg back first in lunge and then your left leg forward on the second lunge. When you've completed a full salutation, try a few more. For a more energizing variation, substitute Warrior 1 (see Chapter 4) for Lunge.

Chapter 4

Standing Tall with Strength and Grace: Standing Poses

Standing poses energize and strengthen the body. They open the hips while increasing power and circulation in the legs, knees, and back. By practicing these asanas, you learn how to embrace your innate strength and tap into your source of power while increasing your balance and courage. Standing poses are the foundation of asana practice, contributing the most postures. The basis for all standing poses is Mountain Pose/Tadasana.

Let's review alignment as it applies to standing poses. Try standing in Mountain Pose/Tadasana, your feet an inch or two apart and parallel. As you inhale, open to receive your fullness, feeling your chest expanding and your heart lifting. We are all stronger and more vibrant than we give ourselves credit for. Keeping your inner brightness, allow your body to soften. Isometrically hug your legs (without moving them) in toward each other. You'll feel your legs engage with muscular energy. Try lifting your toes, feeling your arches, kneecaps, and thighs lifting (more Muscular Energy). Try to keep all this lifted as you release your toes down. Initiate Inner Spiral by slightly turning your thighs in, so the top of your thighs move back and the back of your pelvis widens. As the top of your thighs stay back, tuck your tailbone in Outer Spiral. Now from the core of your pelvis, extend out, stretching your legs. From the rooting down of your legs, there is a natural rising of your heart and extension of your spine. Stand tall with strength and grace.

All standing poses should emphasize the following:

- Muscular Energy to tap into your strength
- Rooting your legs to stay grounded and stable, which allows your nervous system to release
- Opening your hips
- The Pelvic Focal Point

We should all practice standing postures, but they are especially good for those with sedentary jobs, particularly those who spend long hours sitting at a desk or a computer. If you're dealing with emotions of inadequacy, shyness, or feelings of weakness, standing poses can help you shift to being confident and in your power. People with knee, back, and hip issues should also include many standing poses in their routine.

Be Mindful

Before you get in to the standing poses in this chapter, keep the following in mind for all wide-legged standing poses:

Knee awareness: Adjust your stance so your knee is directly over your ankle. If you are too narrow, your knee will go past your ankle, and if you are too wide, your knee will be too far away. Watch that the center of your knee is in line with your second toe. If you tend to hyperextend, spread your toes and actively lift your arches. You may also want to slightly bend your back knee.

Back awareness: If your back thigh is pushing forward, this creates stress on your back. Keep your thigh in line with your torso. Be sure your hips are level and not twisted.

For all balance poses: When practicing balance poses, it is helpful to balance your Muscular and Organic Energy. Think of the sun—it draws particles into its core, charging itself. As it draws in fuel, it can radiate out more light. It is important to root your standing leg.

If you are pregnant: Avoid all poses that constrict your belly. You may want to use a prop, such as a wall, when practicing balance postures. Work with an experienced and certified teacher for other modifications.

Mountain/Tadasana with Arms Extended—Hastasana

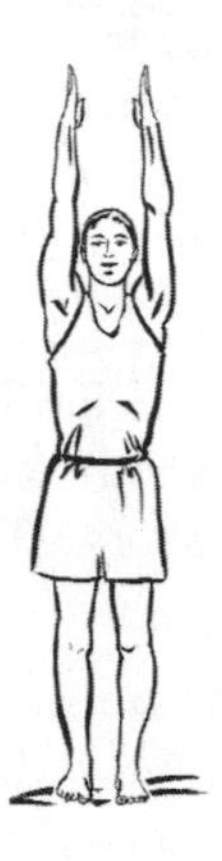

1. Stand with your feet an inch or 2 apart and parallel. When you align physically, you align with your intention.
2. Draw energetically from your feet up toward your pelvis.
3. Keeping your muscles actively engaging, scoop your tailbone and extend energy down through your feet.
4. Continue pressing the four corners of each foot down as you stretch your arms over your head. Notice how everything lifts energetically.
5. Keep extending up as you root down again. Hold for a five deep breaths (30 seconds) to one minute.

Warrior II/Virabhadrasana II

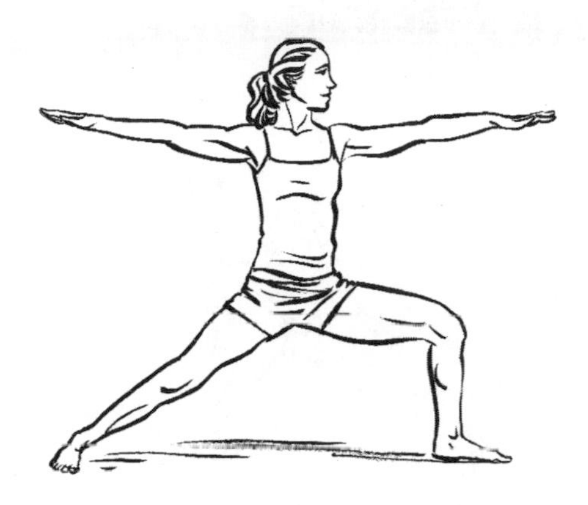

1. Turn lengthwise on your mat, standing with your legs wide apart and your feet parallel.
2. Extend your arms out to T position. Your ankles should be under your wrists.
3. Turn your right toes out 90 degrees and your left in 15 degrees.
4. Inhaling, feel the Prana charging your entire body. As you exhale, bend your right knee over your right ankle. With your next inhalation, draw in from your feet into the core of your pelvis and from your fingers into your heart, embracing your innate strength. Offer that strength out, just as much as you are receiving it.
5. Drop your left hip so it's level with your right.
6. Hold for at least five deep breaths or longer. Repeat on the left side.

Reverse Warrior II/ Reverse Virabhadrasana II

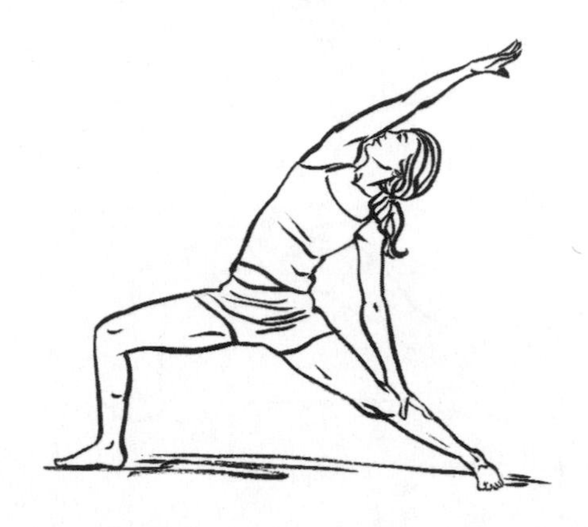

1. In Warrior II, drop your left (straight leg) hand to your thigh and inhale your right (bent knee side) arm up.
2. Plug into your power, drawing your legs into your pelvic focal point. Draw from your fingers into your heart to keep your shoulder drawing into its socket.
3. Exhale as you extend from the pelvis out, rooting your feet. Extend your arm up and over as you slide your left hand down your left thigh. Remember to keep your shoulder blades flat on your back as your heart radiantly opens. Don't lose the bend of your knee.
4. Take at least five deep breaths (or more) and come back into Warrior II. Release and repeat on the opposite side.

Extended Side Angle Variation/ Utthita Parsvakonasana

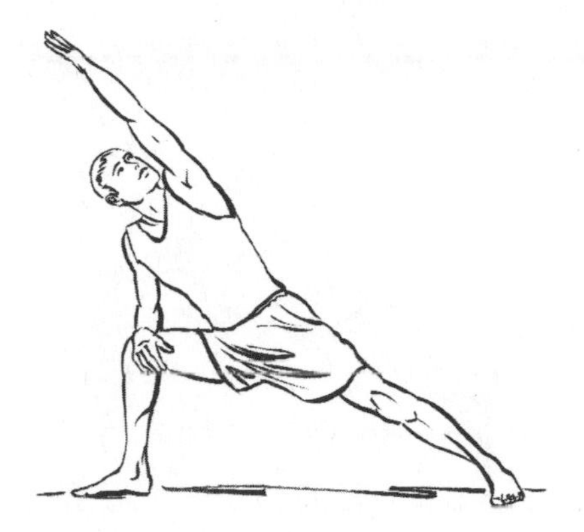

1. From Warrior II, place your right forearm onto your right (bent leg) thigh.
2. Slide your left arm up the side of your body and head, extending your arm to create one long line of energy from your foot to your fingertips.
3. As you inhale, draw from your fingers into the core of your heart and from your legs up into your pelvis, aligning with your strength.
4. Without losing this integration, celebrate this strength by extending out like the rays of the sun. From your left hip root your left foot, lift your lower belly up and away from your left thigh and lengthen you right side body extending out through your crown.
5. Hold for a five breaths to one minute, come back up into Warrior II and the release. Try this asana on the left side.

Extended Side Angle/ Utthita Parsvakonasana

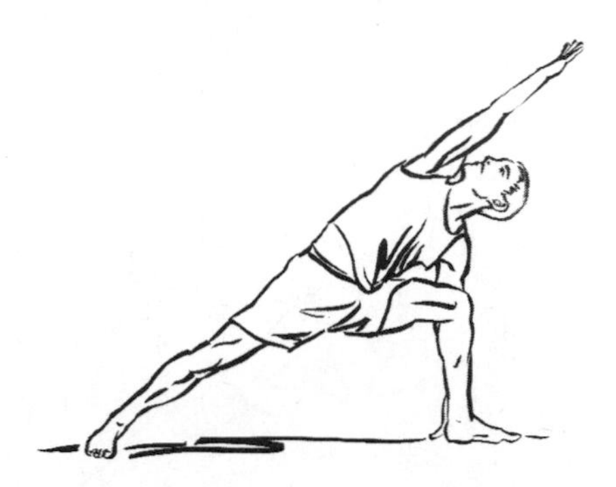

1. Open to receive the fullness of your breath.
2. From Extended Side Angle Variation, place your right hand (bent knee side) on the floor behind your right thigh. Your hand should be directly under your shoulder.
3. Touch just your fingertips to the floor, turning your palm inward to face your leg. Make a strong container out of your body for this Shakti by hugging your legs in.
4. Press your wrist into your shin and your shin into your wrist to charge the pose with more energy.
5. With gratitude for this fullness, extend from your pelvis out your legs, rooting your feet. Make one line of energy from your left foot out through your left fingers.
6. Hold for at least five deep breaths. Repeat on the other side.

Extended Triangle/Utthita Trikonasana

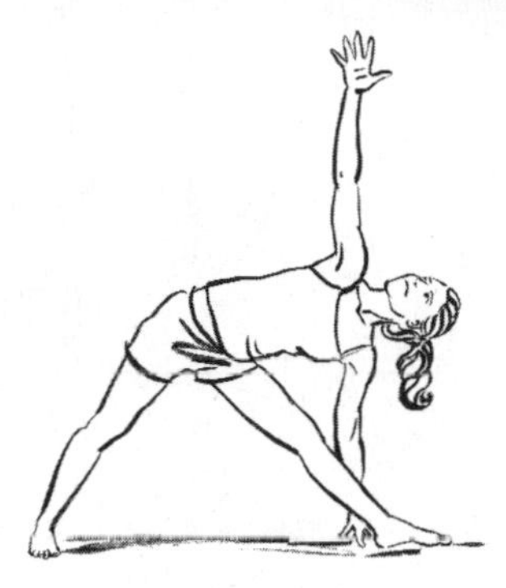

1. Stand lengthwise on your mat, your legs wide apart and your feet parallel. Extend your arms out to T position. Turn your right toes out 90 degrees and your left in 15 degrees.
2. As you inhale, open to the breath that connects you to all things and swell from the inside out. Keeping your connection to something bigger, soften your skin. Draw your legs in and up into the core of your pelvis.
3. Pour yourself over your right leg, placing your right hand on the floor behind your leg or resting your hand on your ankle or shin. Your left arm extends up to the sky.
4. With your exhalation, from your pelvis, root your left foot, and extend out through your crown, lengthening your right side. Be mindful not to hyperextend your knees.
5. Try this pose for five breaths to one minute. Repeat on your left side.

Half Moon/Ardha Chandrasana

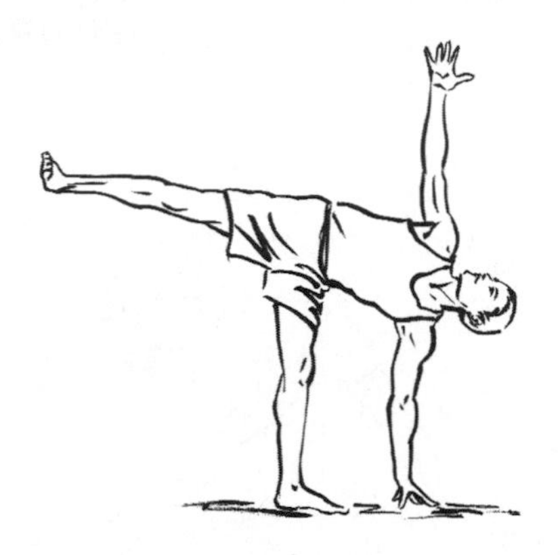

1. From Extended Triangle, bend your right knee, placing your right hand on the floor 1 foot forward of your foot (you may have to step your back foot in to get this important hand spacing). Your left hand can rest on your hip.
2. Shifting your weight onto your right foot, step your left foot in and lift it up so it's parallel to the floor. Straighten your right leg.
3. As you inhale, align with something bigger, and draw from your feet into your pelvis. Both legs stay straight as you stack your hips.
4. As you exhale, from your pelvis extend out through your legs, "stepping" on the back wall and rooting your foundation into the earth.
5. Stretch your left arm up to the sky.
6. Hold for a few breaths or longer before releasing. Repeat on your left side. If you have difficulty balancing, try practicing this pose with your back against the wall.

Sugar Cane Stick/ Ardha Chandra Chipasana

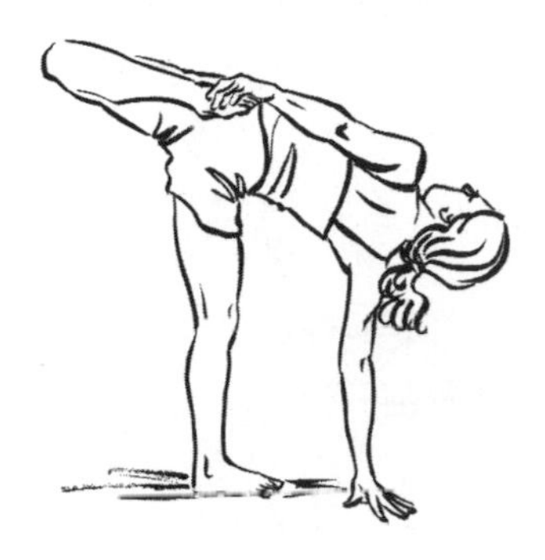

1. From Half Moon, bend your left leg that's lifted into the air and grasp onto your foot behind you with your left hand.
2. Press your foot back into your hand as you open your chest in a backbend.
3. Charge your legs, hugging them in for more stability. The more you stand with strength, rooting your base leg and kicking back, the more you can gracefully bend backward, offering out your heart's desire.
4. Can you hold it for a few breaths or longer? Try it on your other side.

Standing Squat/Utkatasana

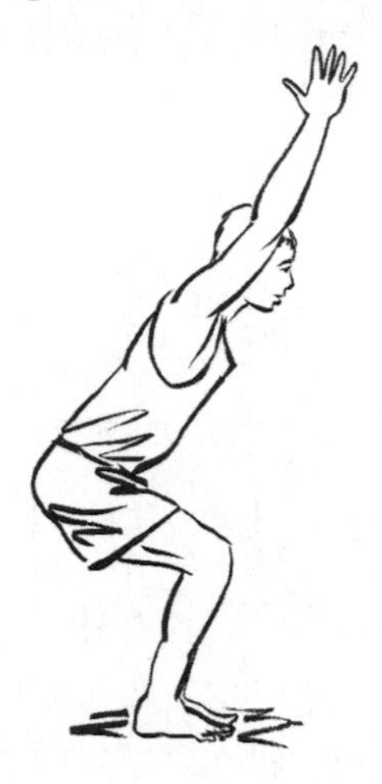

1. Stand in Mountain Pose with your big toes touching so your legs are together.
2. As you inhale, open to receive your true essence. As you exhale, keep this fullness and soften, folding into Forward Bend.
3. Bend your knees so your buttocks are level with the floor. Press your legs into each other in a self-embrace.
4. Walk your fingertips along the floor until your arms are long. Have your palms facing each other. Without moving your legs, lift your chest and head, sweeping your arms overhead, offering back out.
5. Be sure you're not overarching your back. Your tailbone should be pointing down. Hold for five breaths to one minute.

Warrior I Variation/ Virabhadrasana I

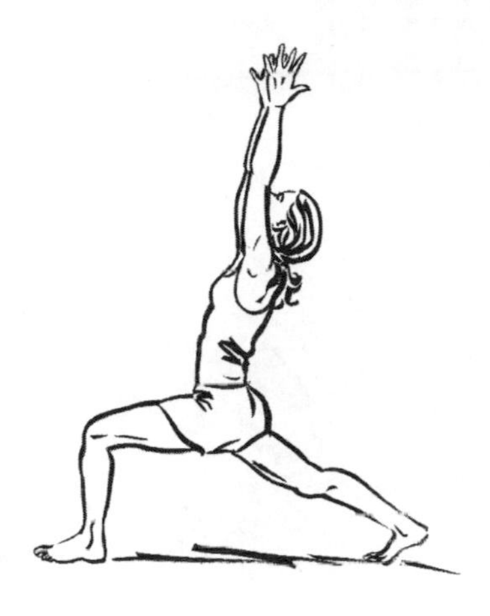

1. From Lunge, place your hands on your hips and come up to standing. Your right (front leg) knee should be over your right ankle, and your left heel (back leg) should be off the floor.
2. Embrace your strength, and draw in from your legs into your pelvis. Reach your left hip forward, and pull your right hip back so your right buttock cheek tucks under and your hips are square.
3. As you inhale, extend your arms overhead. Extend out through your back heel as you reach your left hip forward. Let your arms be a radiant expression of your heart.
4. Enjoy the pose and your breath for a minimum of five breaths. Try Warrior I again with your left leg forward.

Rotated Extended Side Angle Prep/ Parivrtta Utthita Parsvakonasana Prep

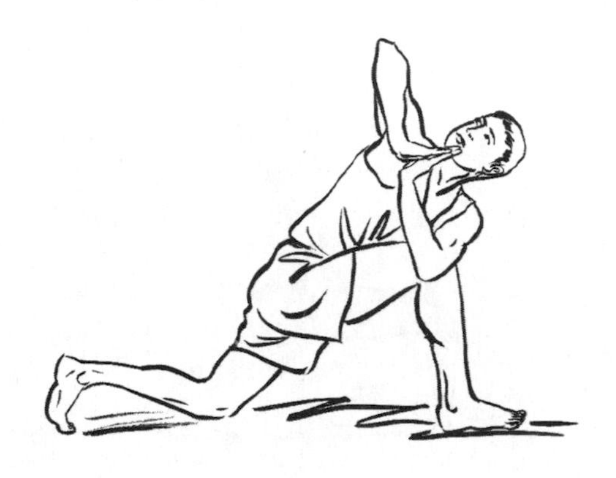

1. Come into Lunge, resting your back (left) knee on the floor.
2. Place your hands on your hips, and sit up tall. Align with pulsation, hug your legs in, and reach your left hip forward while widening out your left buttock out to the left. Your right hip crease pulls back and down, squaring off your hips. Open to receive the energy that feeds all things.
3. Extend your left arm up to the sky, and channel even more breath into your left lung. Keeping this inflation, place your left elbow to the right of your right thigh and bring your hands together in Anjali Mudra (prayer position).

4. Without twisting your hips, with your exhalation, turn your chest to the right and look over your right shoulder. If this is too deep, try placing your forearm on your thigh instead.
5. With your next inhalation, recharge your legs, hugging them in.
6. As you exhale, give thanks, extending from your pelvis out through your heart. Your lower belly will lift in and up as your chest lifts. Hold your pose from 30 seconds to one minute before releasing.

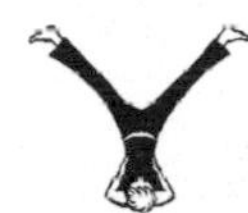

Yoga Speak

All rotated poses are twists. In a true twist, one part stays fixed while the other part moves. (In this pose, your hips stay facing forward as you twist your chest.) That way there is a "wringing" as toxins are squeezed out, and upon release, new blood flushes the area. If you feel that your twist is too deep or you are collapsing your chest toward your thigh, try modifying the pose by placing your forearm on your thigh instead of Anjali Mudra.

Rotated Extended Side Angle/ Parivrtta Utthita Parsvakonasana

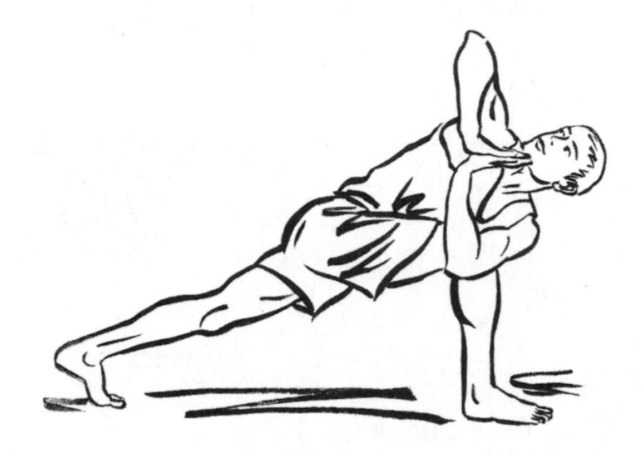

1. From Rotated Extended Side Angle Prep, lift your back knee away from the floor, straightening out, but not hyperextending your leg.
2. With your inhalation, energetically draw in your legs. As you exhale, make this pose a celebration, extending your left heel back toward the earth as your left hip reaches forward and your heart shines out.

Extreme Side Stretch/ Parsvottanasana

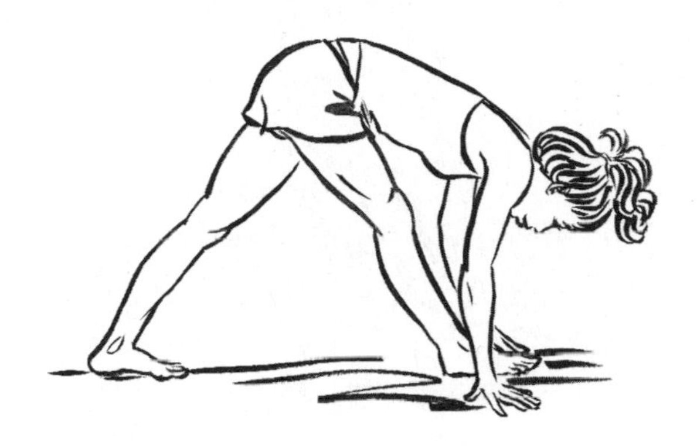

1. Standing in Mountain Pose/Tadasana, step your right foot 3 feet forward. Adjust your width so your back heel remains on the floor.
2. Isometrically hug your legs in toward each other. Reach your left hip forward, and pull your right hip crease back and down to square off your hips.
3. Open to your breath, and bow forward, lengthening your spine.
4. Place your hands on the floor on either side of your right foot. If you can't reach, place your hands on your shin or ankle.
5. Keep your shoulder blades flat on your back as your heart reaches out its desire for absolute freedom forward. Be mindful not to hyperextend your knees.
6. Try holding this for at least five full breaths before releasing. Repeat on the opposite side.

Rotated Extended Triangle/ Parivrtta Utthita Trikonasana

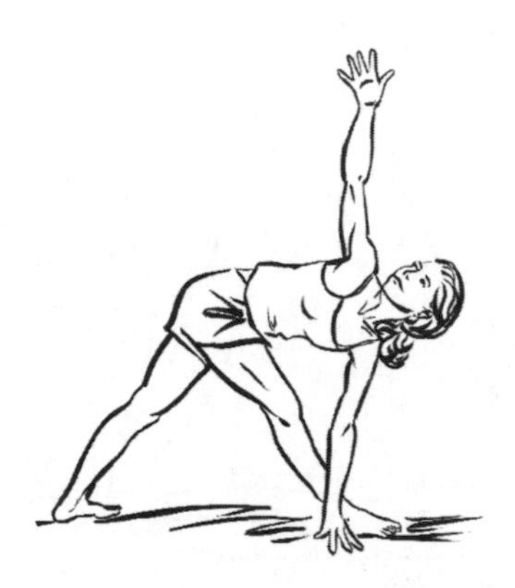

1. From Extended Side Angle, place your right hand on your right hip and move your left hand to the right of your right ankle. If you place just your fingertips on the floor and turn your palm facing your leg, you can press your wrist into your shin and access more leg strength.
2. Turn and look over your right shoulder. As you twist, rather than rotate, initiate the twist by moving from the back of your left ribs over to the right while keeping your left hip up so your hips stay even in height.
3. Keep reaching your left hip forward and drawing your right hip crease back as you deepen the twist. Breathe into your left kidney, expanding it up to the sky so your left hip doesn't drop.
4. Now extend your right arm up to the sky. Hold for five or more breaths and then repeat on the other side.

Rotated Half Moon/ Parivrtta Ardha Chandrasana

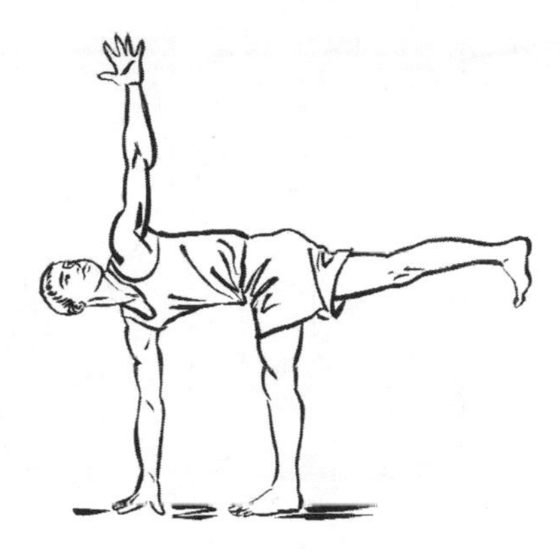

1. From Rotated Extended Triangle, place your right hand on your right hip and bend your right knee. Keeping your left hand to the right of your right foot, move it about 10 inches forward.
2. Shift your weight onto your right foot as you extend your left leg back.
3. Straighten both legs as you stand with strength.
4. Inhale and draw from your feet into your pelvis, charging your core just like the sun.
5. If you're really stable, exhale and open your chest to the right, extending your right arm up to the sky.
6. Make your arms and legs as radiant as the sun. From your core, extend out. Even your toes sparkle as they spread out for extra balance.
7. Can you hold for five deep breaths? Repeat on left side.

Standing Split/ Urdhva Prasarita Ekapadasana

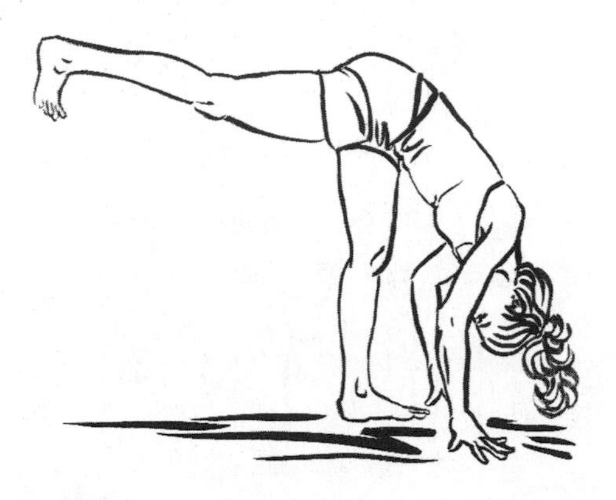

1. Place your fingertips on the floor in Standing Forward Bend.
2. How much do you want your intention? Draw this ideal in, drawing your legs in and up into your pelvis.
3. Shift your weight onto your right leg, and extend your left leg up toward the sky. Looking back at your left toes, make your pinky toe and big toe level so your hip is not turning out.
4. Keeping both legs straight, bow to this ideal, folding forward. Try lifting your right toes up to activate your leg.
5. Lengthen your legs, pressing the four corners of your standing foot into the earth.
6. Hold for a few breaths. After you release the first side, try lifting the right leg.

Warrior III/Virabhadrasana III

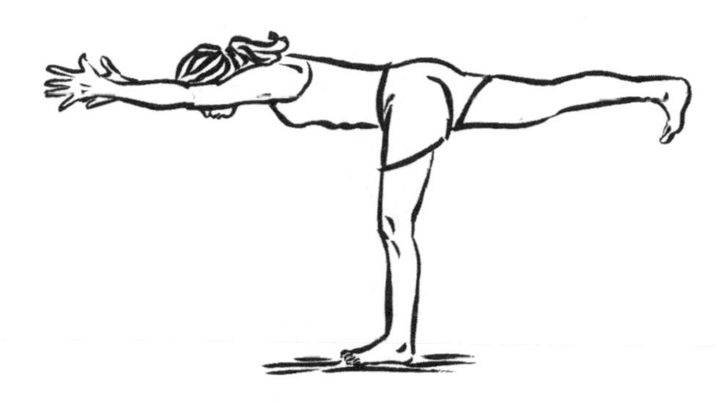

1. From Standing Split, bring your leg parallel to the floor and lift your hands off the floor, extending your arms forward. (You may find it easier to enter Warrior III through a standing position.)
2. Create more fullness in this moment by hugging in your legs.
3. While staying engaged, extend from your legs out, rooting your standing leg down. Offer out 100 percent.
4. Can you hold for five full breaths? Longer? Repeat on left.

Warrior I/Virabhadrasana I

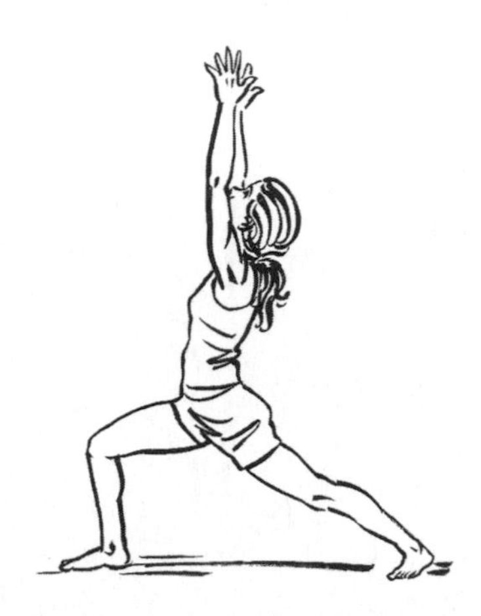

1. From Mountain Pose/Tadasana, step your right foot forward, bending your right knee over your right ankle. In the full version of this pose (see Warrior I Variation), your back foot is completely grounded. If your back foot is parallel to the wall behind you, turn your toes slightly in, as it will be easier to square off your hips.
2. Drawing your feet in toward each other and up into your pelvis, reach your left hip forward. As you line up physically, you align with your intention.
3. Balance hugging in with extending out from your pelvis through your feet, pressing them into the earth. Extend your arms up to the sky, reaching out that desire.
4. Hold this pose for 30 seconds to 1 minute. Don't forget to do Warrior I on the other side.

Wide-Legged Forward Bend with Hands Clasped Behind the Back/ Prasarita Padottanasana

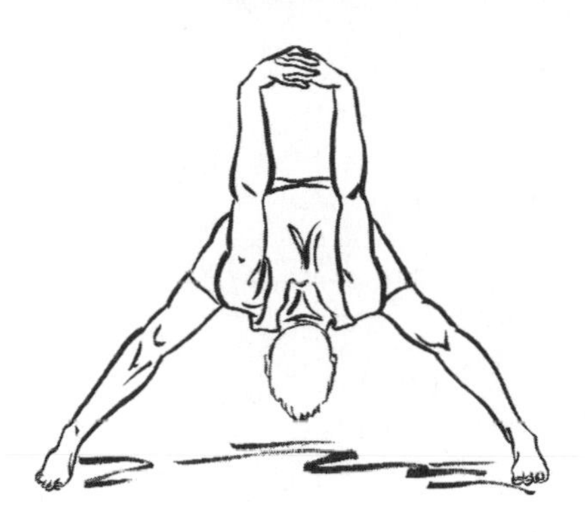

1. Stand with your legs wide apart and your feet parallel. As you inhale, your heart and lungs expanding, let your arms ride the wave of your breath, interlacing your fingers behind you, palms facing each other.
2. Isometrically hug your legs in toward each other. Turn your thighs slightly in and back so your buttocks widen behind you.
3. Keeping the top of your thighs back, scoop your tailbone and extend through your legs into your feet.
4. Let your heart lead the way as you bow forward, honoring your uniqueness, stretching your arms away from your back.
5. Enjoy your breath fully, holding the pose for five breaths or longer.

Tree Pose/Vrksasana

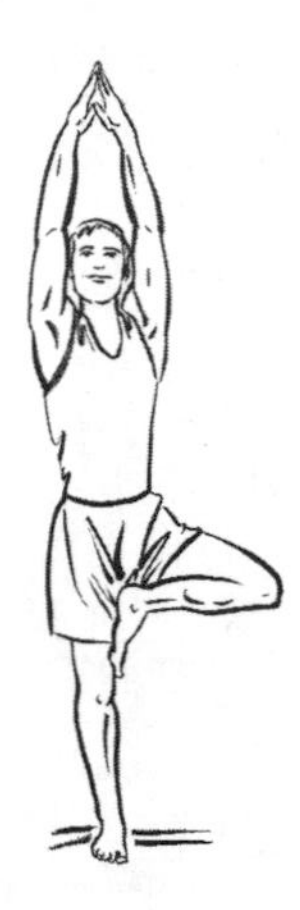

1. Standing in Mountain Pose/Tadasana, shift your weight onto your right foot and place your left foot against your inner right thigh. Alternatively, you can have your foot lower, even at your ankle, just don't press on your inner knee.
2. Awaken your stability, press your foot into your leg and leg into your foot.
3. Place your hands in Anjali Mudra and extend your intention out your arms lengthening up to the sky.
4. From your pelvis, root your standing leg, pressing the four corners of your foot into the earth. If you're having trouble balancing, hold your arms out in T position, like a tight-rope walker. It's helpful to softly gaze at a fixed point on the wall or horizon.
5. Try balancing for at least five full breaths and repeat on the other side.

Eagle/Garudasana

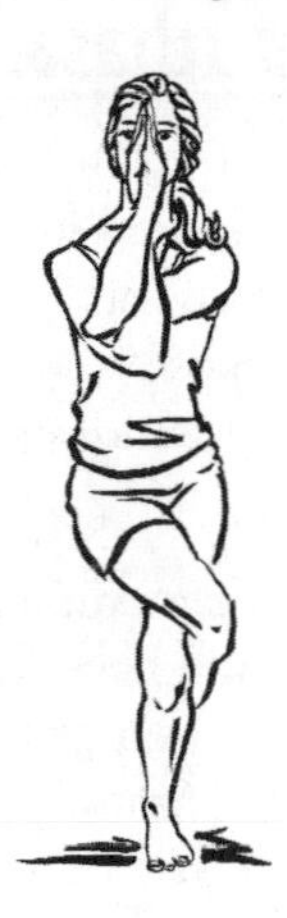

1. Stand in Mountain Pose/Tadasana. As you inhale, bring your arms out to shoulder height and then hug yourself so your right arm is under your left.
2. Keeping your elbows stacked, wrap your forearms around each other, bringing your hands together as close as possible.
3. Shift your weight onto your left foot, and cross your right leg over your left. If you can, tuck your right toes behind your left leg. Draw your legs together in a self-embrace. This is part one of the pose and may be challenging enough.
4. For part two, bend your knees as you come into a squat with your buttocks parallel to the floor. Without losing your engagement, can you soften into this moment?
5. Can you hold for a few breaths or more? Repeat Eagle on your other side.

Hand to Big Toe Series/ Hasta Padangusthasana

Each part of the Hand to Big Toe Series can be done by itself or integrated in a flow. Feel free to take a break in between each pose and work up to flowing from one pose to the next. If you have trouble balancing, try standing with your back against a wall.

This series can also be modified to do lying on your back. (In Part III, you'll have to cross over your leg instead of twisting your chest.) To protect your back, keep the inner thigh of your standing leg back. (This is the one you're not moving if you're practicing this pose on the floor.)

Try holding each pose for at least five deep breaths or longer.

Hand to Big Toe Series—Part I

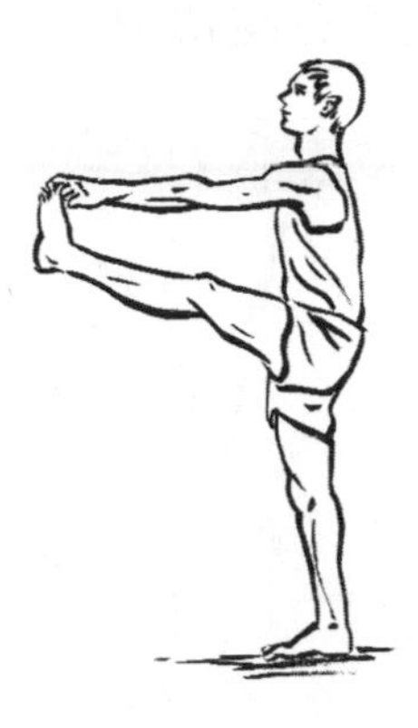

1. Begin standing in Mountain Pose/Tadasana. Shifting your weight onto your right foot, bend your left knee into your chest.
2. Place a strap around your left foot or grasp onto your left big toe with your left hand. If you're using a strap, place your hands on each end of the strap. If you're using your hand, rest your right hand on your hip.
3. Create balance in your life by cultivating balance in this moment. To support this, hug your legs in, embracing stability.
4. Keeping your hips level, stretch your left leg straight. Stand up tall, avoid leaning back to counterbalance. (It is great to practice this while keeping your back against a wall or lying on your back.)
5. With your hand or strap, pull the foot in and extend from your foot back out. Are your shoulder blades flat on your back?

Hand to Big Toe Series—Part II: To Side

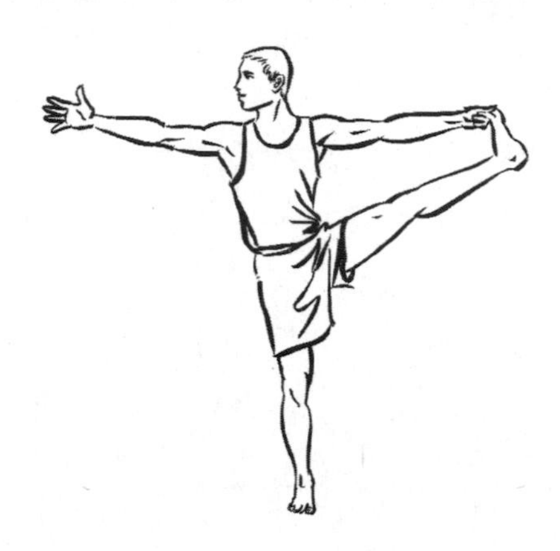

1. From Part I, switch the strap ends into your left hand (or keep holding onto your toe).
2. Open your leg out to the left. Be mindful that you're not leaning to the right to counterbalance.
3. Stand up tall and proud, keeping the hips level. Spread your toes. Maintain a balance of receiving (drawing your legs in) and offering (extending your legs out).
4. If you want to create more challenge, extend your right arm to the right and softly gaze at your fingertips.

Hand to Big Toe Series—Part III: Rotated

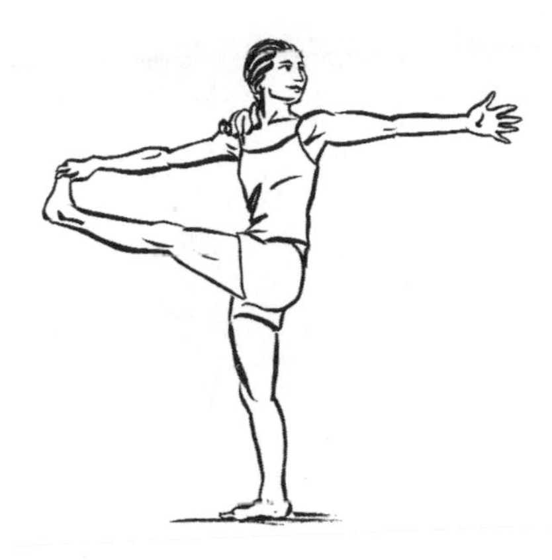

1. From Part II, bring your leg back to center. Switch your strap ends to your right hand. If you were holding onto your toe, hold onto the left side of your foot with your right hand.
2. Plug into your birthright, aligning with your strength, and draw from your feet into your pelvis.
3. Leaving your left leg forward, with your exhalation, turn and twist your chest open to the left. You can extend your left arm behind you and look at the fingertips.
4. Extend from your pelvis back out through your feet, pressing one into the floor and the other into your hand. The more stability you have in your legs, the more you can open your chest wholeheartedly and twist.

Hand to Big Toe Series—Part IV

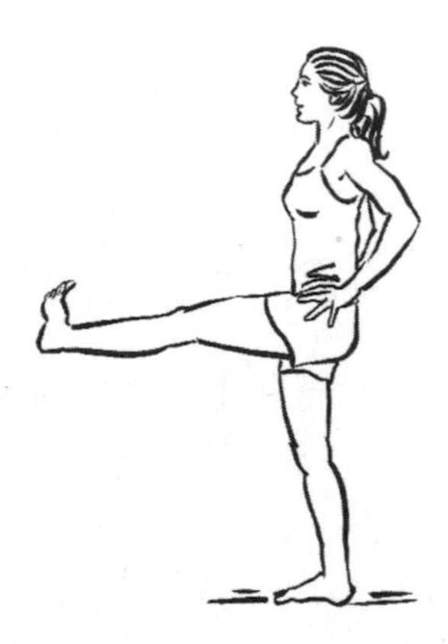

1. If you're continuing from Part III, bring your leg back to center. If you're doing this by itself, follow Part I.
2. Release your hands or strap from your foot, and try to keep your leg extended.
3. Create a strong container out of your body to channel Prana, drawing your legs into your pelvis. Offer your power back out to this larger force, extending out through your legs, rooting your standing leg. Even your toes spread out enthusiastically.

Chapter 5

Blossoming the Lotus: Hip Openers and Quad Stretches

The hips are a common place for tension to collect. As the hips tighten, so do the muscles around the hips, leading to back and leg problems. As the thigh muscles tighten, so do the hips and lower back. Keeping the hips and thighs open is crucial to a healthy back. As the hips release their tension, circulation returns to its optimal flow, nourishing the reproductive organs and the spine. The energy of release, *Apana Vayu*, flows downward, allowing the nervous system to calm and the digestive and eliminatory systems to balance. This energy returning to the earth has a calming, stabilizing, and quieting effect.

Having the proper alignment in the hips helps them open. It's a common mistake to practice hip openers passively, which tightens the muscles after they initially stretch. To truly open your hips, you must stay engaged, like a lotus flower rooting into the mud.

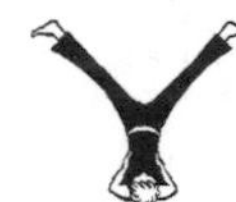

Yoga Speak

One of the five main Pranas, **Apana Vayu** is downward flowing. It governs the area from the navel down, assisting with elimination, reproduction, and digestion. Try a sighing exhalation, and you'll feel the releasing effects of Apana Vayu on the nervous system.

Follow these alignment steps to allow your hips to blossom open:

Charge your legs with muscular energy. Hugging your legs in toward each other, draw from your feet into your pelvis.

Activate Inner Spiral, turning your thighs slightly in toward each other and moving the top of your thighs back, widening your back thighs apart as the back of your pelvis broadens.

Add Outer Spiral by scooping your tailbone, rooting it down toward the earth. From your pelvis, lengthen your legs.

Try to keep your hips square and even so they remain level. (Don't move so deeply that you lose the alignment.)

Be mindful not to overstretch. Do not open your hips passively, as this creates more tension later. Keep drawing your legs into the pelvic focal point to stay engaged.

If you're pregnant, avoid any poses in which your womb presses into the floor or your body.

Knee Down Lunge/Anjaneyasana

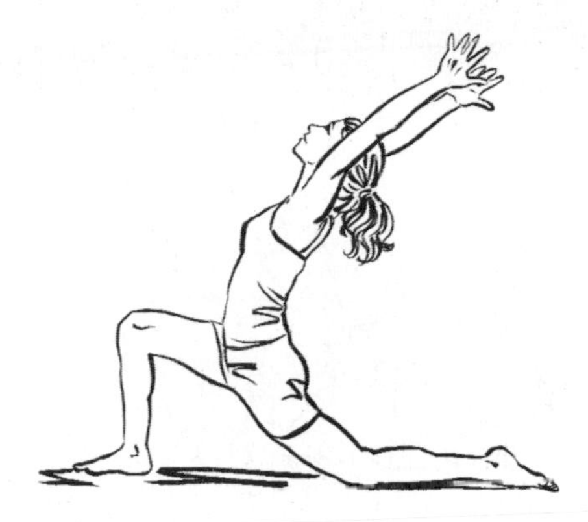

1. Coming onto all fours, step your right foot forward in between your hands.
2. Slide your left knee back so you're resting the top of your kneecap on the floor. (This will help take the pressure off your knee. If it still doesn't relieve the pressure, try using extra padding under your knee.)
3. Inhale your arms over your head.
4. Establish your roots, drawing your legs in and up into the pelvis. The left hip reaches forward, your left buttock widens out to the left, while your right hip crease moves back and down.
5. Maintain the hugging-in (muscles engaged) as you bend your right knee a bit more and lower your inner left thigh toward the floor.
6. Keep feeding your roots as you extend your arms over your head, lifting and expanding your heart so it fully blossoms.
7. Stay in this pose for at least five breaths. Repeat with your left leg forward.

Knee Down Lunge with Quad Stretch

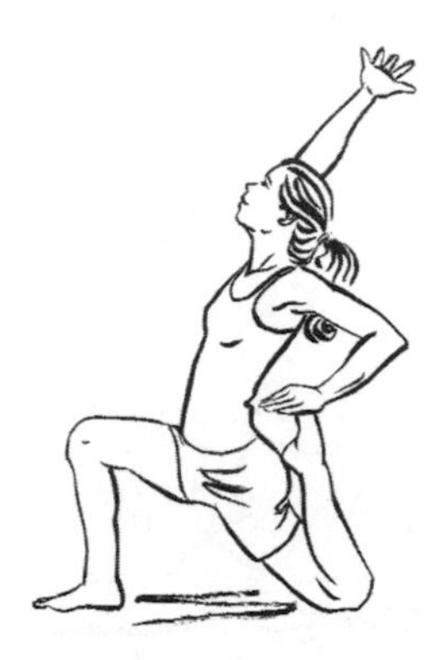

1. From Knee Down Lunge, lift your left foot away from the floor until you feel a stretch. If your thigh is tight, lifting it up a few inches may be enough. You may need to grasp onto the foot and pull your heel into your buttocks.
2. Hug your legs in, and create more engagement by pressing your foot back into your hand. Keep reaching your left hip forward and pulling your right buttocks back and down.
3. With your next inhalation, open to receive your inherent fullness. Your pelvis will lift slightly away from the floor.
4. Keeping your brightness, as you exhale, soften your skin and come deeper into the pose, lowering your inner left thigh a bit more. Be sure your hips stay level.
5. Soften into your effort as you hold this pose for a few breaths. Repeat on other side.

Sphinx

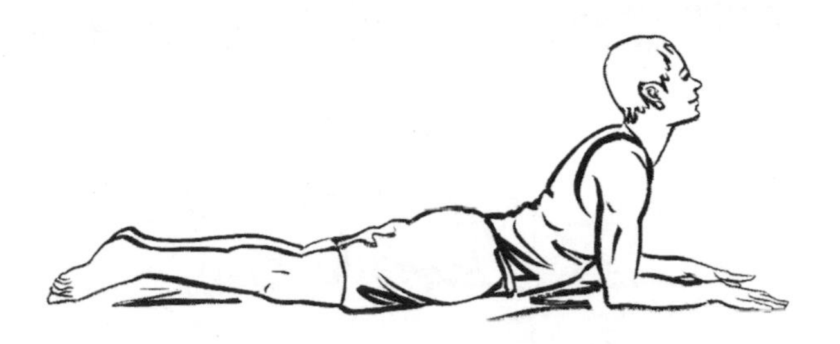

1. Lying on your belly, place your hands on the floor under your shoulders.
2. Hug your shins in and down as you scoop your tailbone toward your toes.
3. Slide your hands forward so you're resting on your forearms and your elbows are directly under your shoulders. You are now propped up on your arms so your chest is lifted.
4. Embrace your power, plugging in from your toes into your pelvis and claw the floor (drawing your fingers energetically toward your heart).
5. As you hug in, create an offering extend out, lifting and expanding your heart and lengthening your leg bones.
6. Enjoy your breath a few more times before releasing.

Half Frog/Ardha Bhekasana

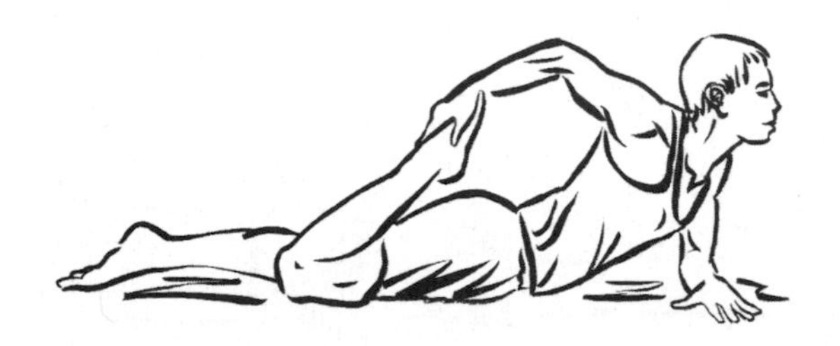

1. From Sphinx, turn your right forearm in so it's parallel to your waist line.
2. Bend your left knee, moving your heel toward your buttocks, until you feel the stretch in your thigh. You may need to grasp onto your foot and pull your heel into your buttocks. Create resistance by pressing the foot back into the hand.
3. It's a common misalignment to twist in this pose. Align with your intention by reaching the left side of your chest forward.
4. Draw your shoulder blades onto the back of your heart, feeding your heart's desire.
5. Continue in the pose for a few more breaths. Release and try on the right side.

Pigeon Prep/ Eka Pada Rajakapotasana Prep

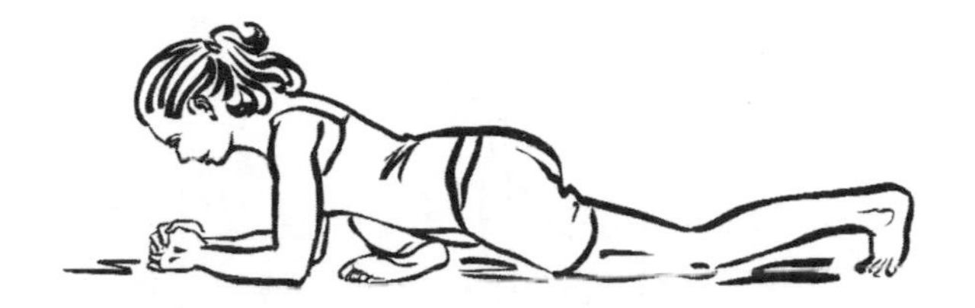

1. On all fours, slide your right knee in between your hands and extend your left leg straight back.
2. Move your right knee slightly out toward your right hand and right toes a bit toward your left hand. (The more flexible you are, the more your shin can come parallel to your waist line.) Be sure your left leg is straight back and that you curl your toes under.
3. Channel your power, hug your legs in, and you'll feel your pelvis lift away from the floor.
4. Turn your thighs slightly in toward each other, back, and apart so your buttocks widen behind you.
5. Scoop your tailbone as you bow in self-honoring, hinging at your hips. Keep moving your left hip forward and your right hip crease back and down.
6. Hold this for at least five breaths. Don't forget to do the pose on the other side.

Half Pigeon/ Eka Pada Rajakapotasana

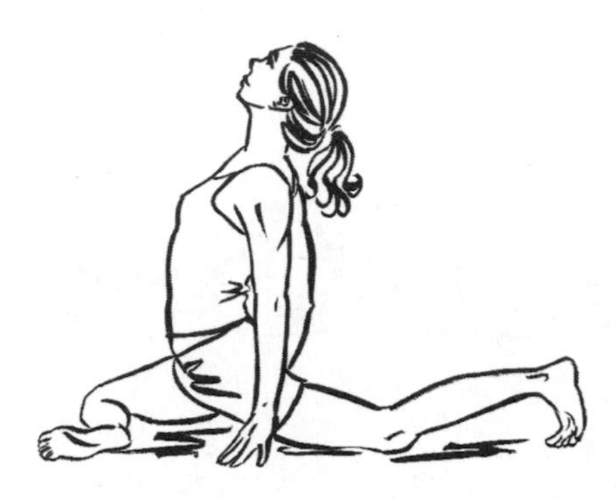

1. From Pigeon Prep, slide your cup shaped hands (fingertips) on the earth under your shoulders.
2. Lift your chest with a Cobra back, leading from your heart. Slide your hands as close into your hips as possible. Draw into your core, from your legs into your pelvis.
3. Reach your left hip forward and your right hip crease back, squaring your hips. Scoop your tailbone.
4. Inhaling, take the top of your ears back so your neck is in line with your spine. Keeping your lungs inflated, draw your shoulder blades onto your back. Your heart unfolds like a blossom, offering out its unique beauty. Maintaining the lift of your heart, soften your shoulder blades.
5. Take a few more deep breaths. Repeat on the other side.

Full Frog Variation/Bhekasana

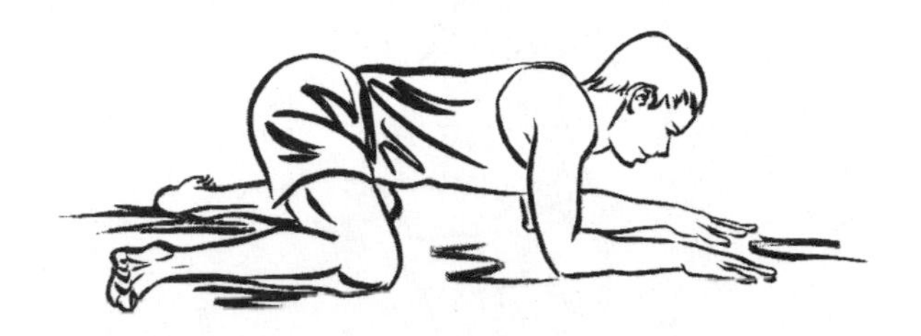

1. Come onto all fours, knees about 1 foot wider than hip-width apart.
2. Flex your feet. Because your shins tend to drop in, be sure the angle between your calves and thighs is 90 degrees.
3. Come down onto your forearms. As you inhale, your whole body surges with Prana. Energetically, hug your legs in, making a strong container for this Shakti.
4. Turn your thighs slightly in and back, and scoop your tailbone.
5. With your exhalation, tension drops away as your skin softens.
6. Rock your hips forward and back. If you don't feel a stretch, take your knees wider apart. Once you feel something, press your buttocks back, holding the stretch for five or more deep breaths.

Baby Cradle

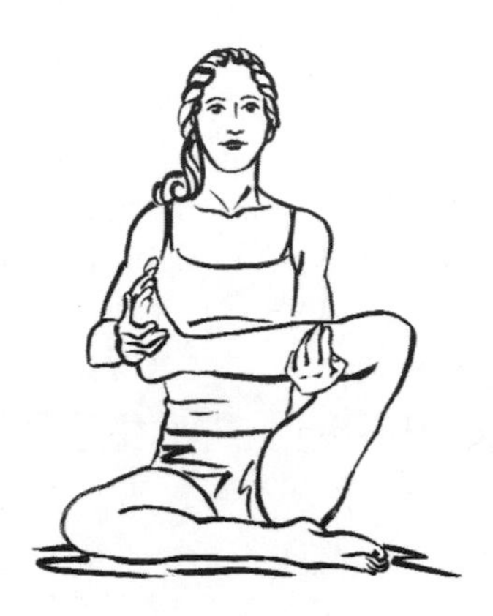

1. Sit up tall in Simple Seated Pose. If your lower back collapses or your knees are higher than your hips, sit on a blanket.
2. Hold on to one leg, bringing your calf parallel to your body. Hold your leg in a way that allows you to maintain an erect spine. Rock your leg back and forth a few times as if you are cradling a baby.
3. Come into stillness. You want your life to blossom? Move within, plugging your legs into the pelvis. Press your foot into your hand and your hand into your foot to create additional resistance.
4. As you roll your thighs slightly in toward each other and down, you'll feel your pelvis tilt forward.

5. Scoop your tailbone. From the condensed energy of the darkness within, offer out your light, lift your heart, and lengthen out through your crown.
6. Maintain this engagement as you soften into your breath. Try holding this for a few breaths before repeating on your opposite side.

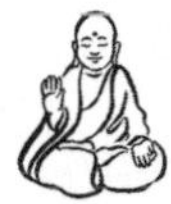

Be Mindful

Hip openers can be intense without creating tension. A sign of tensing is holding in the breath and gripping muscles such as the jaw. Can you engage in the pose and relax into it? Breathe deeply; allow your skin to soften; relax your jaw and tongue by softly smiling.

Bound Angle/Baddha Konasana

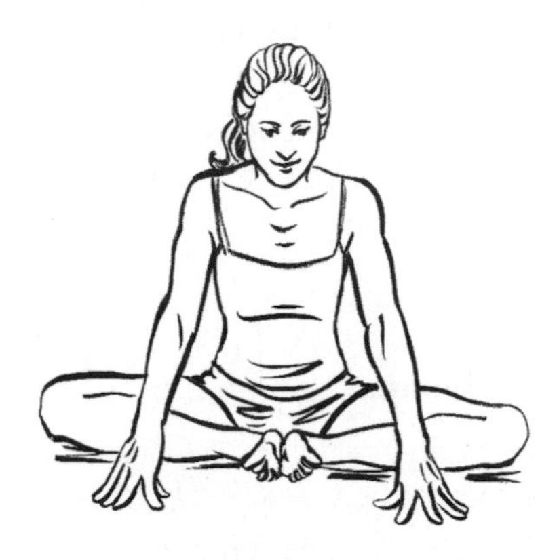

1. Sit up tall, on blankets if necessary, your spine extending in both directions and your hands cup-shaped on the floor by your hips.
2. Place the soles of your feet together and your knees wide apart. If your knees are higher than your hips, raise the height of your blanket.
3. Lift your knees slightly as you press your feet into each other. Align with your intention as you physically line up.
4. Turn your thighs slightly in and down, and your pelvis will tilt forward. Rooting your tailbone down, soften your knees.
5. Repeat a few times. Your knees will drop a little lower each time as your hips open.

Cow Face Legs/Gomukhasana Legs

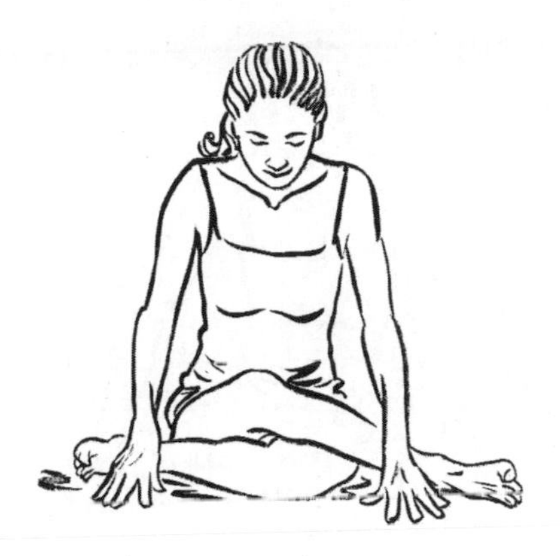

1. From a seated position (sitting up on support if needed) place both feet on the floor.
2. Slide your left foot under your right leg so your foot is by your right hip. Your right knee is centered on your torso.
3. Stack your right leg on top of your left, knee upon knee, so that your right foot is by your left hip. Depending on your hips, this may look very different.
4. Flex both feet. Embracing your strength, hug your legs in as you gently turn your thighs in toward each other and down toward the floor.
5. Keeping the top of your thighs back, scoop your tailbone.
6. Pull your top hip's crease back and down. Bow forward, offering back out as much as you've received.
7. Without losing your engagement, soften into your pose for a few more breaths. Try your second side.

Fire Log Pose/Agnistambhasana

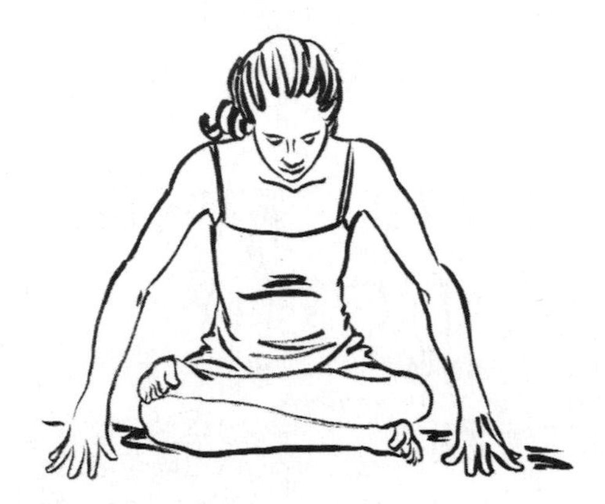

1. Begin in Simple Seated Position (sitting up on support if needed), and place both feet on the floor.
2. Place your left foot under your right leg, touching your whole outer leg to the earth.
3. Bring your calf as parallel to your torso as you can.
4. Stack the other leg on top (as close as possible), flexing your feet. Your legs should resemble stacked firewood.
5. Feed the fire of your intention, drawing your legs in energetically. As you turn your thighs slightly in and down, your pelvis will widen back and apart.
6. Keeping the top of your thighs back, scoop your tailbone and bow forward.
7. To deepen the sensation, draw your right buttocks back and down. This should make you smile.
8. As you hold this pose for a few more breaths, make sure you are not tensing. Repeat on your other side.

Chapter 6

Trusting Your Strength: Hand Balances

Balancing on your hands cultivates strength, focus, integration, and equanimity. Although challenging, these asanas are incredibly energizing and rewarding. When you balance on your hands, you feel alive. You are a strong and vibrant being, playfully exploring gravity.

The key to hand balances is in the alignment of the shoulders and heart. When your shoulder blades are firmly on your back, you can access your back muscles. With three layers, your back muscles are much stronger than your arms. Rounded shoulders cut off Prana to the elbows, wrists, and hands. Weight bearing on your hands with this misalignment can be painful. While the shoulder blades stay flat on the back, the heart can be soft.

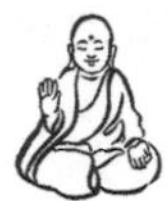

Be Mindful

If you have wrist, hand, elbow, or shoulder injuries, you may want to refrain from doing hand balances. Depending on your condition, you may be able to work with a teacher to practice these poses modified. Sometimes a slight shift in alignment allows you to do these poses pain-free.

Try this exercise to align your shoulders:

1. Feel your breath expanding your whole body as you open to receive your innate strength.
2. Placing a hand behind the base of your head, press your head back into your hand. This aligns your neck with your spine. (Because most of us push our heads forward, this returns the natural curve to the neck.) Keeping the base of your skull over your tailbone, release your hand back down.
3. Breathing into your lungs, expand the sides of your ribs so your shoulders rise up slightly toward your ears.
4. Draw your shoulder blades onto your back so your heart lifts and expands.
5. Keeping the top of your arm up, relax your shoulder blades down.

Another key to hand balancing is the placement of your hands. Like the feet, there are *Four Corners of the Hands* that, when rooted down, help the arch of your palm to lift. The creases of your wrists should be parallel to the front of your mat. Your fingers should be spread out widely, like rays of the sun.

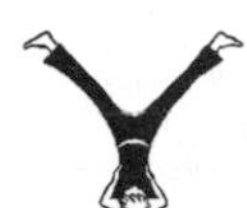

Yoga Speak

When the **Four Corners of the Hands** are rooted, the arch of the palm lifts. Ground the following:

- The fleshy mound between your thumb and your wrist.
- The fleshy mound where your palm meets your index finger.
- The point where your outer wrist meets your hand.
- The base of your pinky finger where it meets your hand.

In this chapter, I have included a preparation pose before each pose. The prep poses are ideal for those just starting out with hand balances. Because these poses are modified, they allow you to work slowly with strength and balance.

I have also included two inversions at the end of the chapter. Inversions are also hand balances. You can find more inversions in Chapter 8.

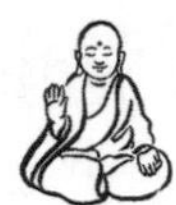

Be Mindful

The last two poses are considered to be inversions as well as hand balances. Inversions are not recommended if you have high blood pressure, a detached retina, are menstruating, or are pregnant and have never done inversions.

Side Plank Prep/Vasisthasana Prep

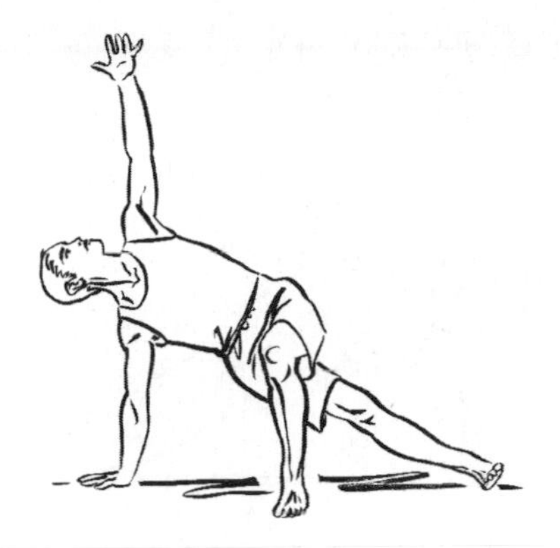

1. Come into Downward Facing Dog. Step your right hand 1 inch toward your left.
2. Come onto the right side of your right foot, so the sole is facing away from you.
3. Bend your left knee, and place your left foot on the floor in front of your belly, toes facing away from you.
4. Plug into your power, drawing from your fingers into your heart. Pressing your right hand, the right side of your foot, and your left foot into the earth, lift your left arm up toward the sky.
5. Lift your hips as you open your heart, celebrating your strength. Try holding this for a few breaths before doing the opposite side.

Side Plank/Vasisthasana

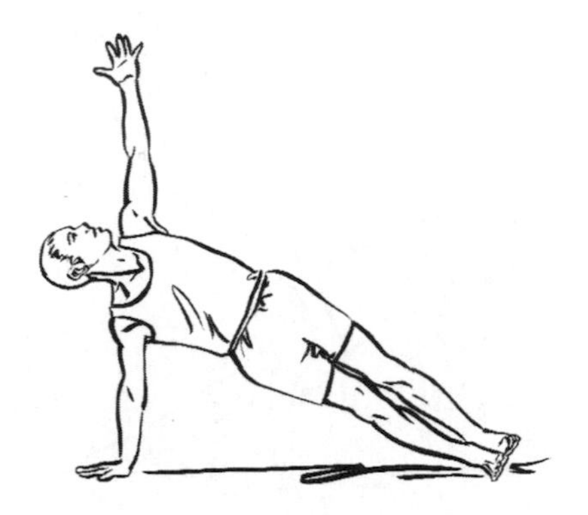

1. Come into Side Plank Prep. Stack your left leg upon your right. Your feet are stacked on top of each other.
2. Draw energetically from your hands and feet into your heart in self-honoring.
3. Keep lifting your hips as you let your arms and legs become a radiant expression of your heart.
4. Try spreading your toes to increase balance, creating a fuller celebration. Can you hold this for a few breaths before trying the other side?

Crane Prep/Bakasana Prep

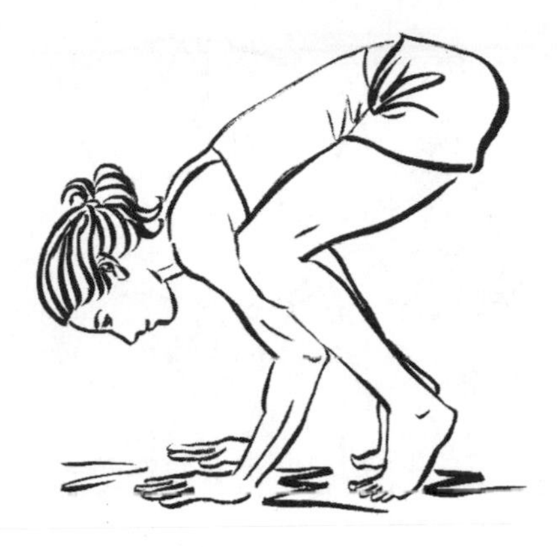

1. With your feet wide apart and parallel, come into a squat.
2. Place your hands on the floor shoulder-width apart. Your heels will come off the earth.
3. Enjoy the gift of your breath. Isometrically swipe your hands in toward each other.
4. With your next inhalation, feel your lungs expanding.
5. Slide your palate back, so your neck is in line with your spine just as it was when you pressed your head into your hand.
6. Draw your shoulder blades firmly on your back. Keeping them there, allow your heart to soften with gratitude toward the floor.
7. Now from your heart, extend your hands back into the earth.

Full Crane/Bakasana

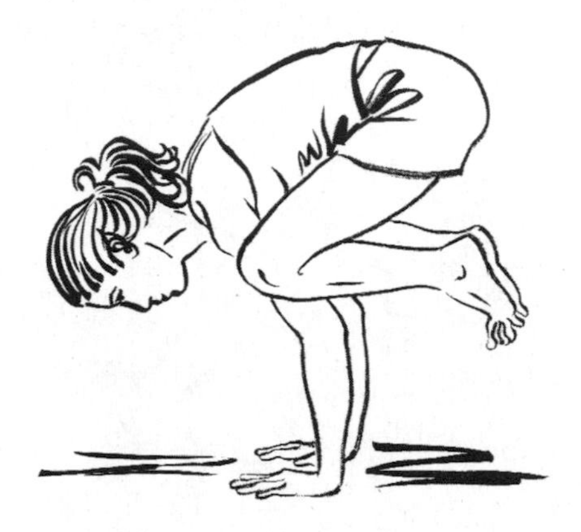

1. From Crane Prep, lift your buttocks into the air. In your essence you are fullness. Align with the bigger flow, drawing your hands energetically in and up into your heart.
2. Without losing your hugging in (engaging), bend your elbows out to the sides, making "shelves" out of your arms.
3. Place your shins on these as you shift your weight forward. It will take practice to be able to take both feet off the floor.
4. Once they're airborne, hug your legs toward each other so you reinforce your arms. Breathe into your lower back, expanding it up, and melt your heart toward the floor.
5. Explore holding this pose and continue to breath deeply.

Handstand Prep/ Ardha Adho Mukha Vrksasana

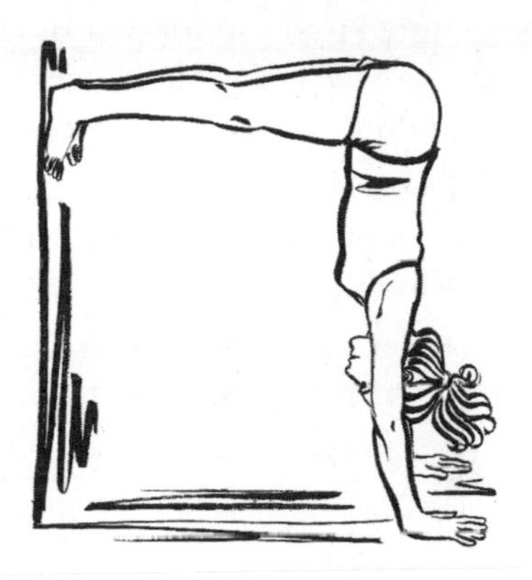

1. Sit with your back against an empty wall, your legs extended in front of you. Mark this area where your heels are and come onto all fours, placing your palms where your feet just were.
2. Observe your breath. Isometrically swipe your hands in and draw from your fingers into your heart. As you plug in, you'll feel your shoulder blades magnetizing on the back of your heart. Keeping this strength and integration, from your heart, extend your power out through your hands.
3. Curl your toes under and press into Downward Facing Dog with your heels on the wall.
4. One foot at a time, step on the wall at the height of your hips. If your legs are higher than your hips, you're making it harder for yourself.

5. Now offer out 100 percent, straighten your legs, and press your heels into the wall. Your hips will come directly over your shoulders. Although you'll be tempted to do so for fear of falling over, *do not walk your hands away!* Your feet are more likely to slide down the wall, which is safer.
6. From your heart, offer back to the source, re-rooting your hands. Keeping your hands in place aligns your shoulders and hips.
7. As your shoulder blades feed the back of your heart, your heart melts with gratitude.

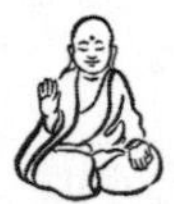

Be Mindful

Both Handstand Prep and Handstand are inversions. Please see the Inversion Cautions in Chapter 8.

Handstand/Adho Mukha Vrksasana (literally: Downward Facing Tree)

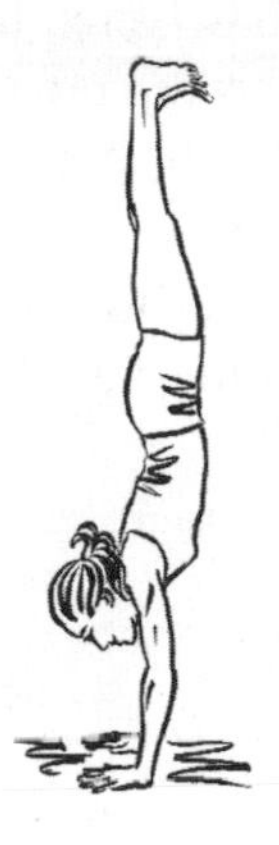

1. Come into Downward Facing Dog while facing an empty wall, your hands one hand's width away from the wall.
2. Isometrically swipe your hands in and draw your hands into your heart. Your shoulder blades will come onto your back. From your heart, extend back out through your hands like stable roots of a tree extending down into the earth.
3. *Be sure you're familiar with hand and shoulder alignment outlined in this chapter before proceeding.*
4. Step one foot in half way, and keep the opposite leg straight.
5. Rooting the Four Corners of the Hands, hop on your bent leg as if you're jumping on a trampoline. Keep the opposite leg absolutely straight. Eventually, the straight leg will rise up to the wall and the other leg will follow.

6. Once you're up, look down at your rooted hands and slide your heels up the wall as a tree freely extends up to the sky.
7. The back tends to overarch here. To remedy this, bend one knee and place your foot against the wall. Draw your belly in as you extend the tailbone up to the sky.
8. Try holding for a few breaths or as long as you can maintain the integrity of the pose.

Hand and Arm Pose/ Eka Hasta Bhujasana

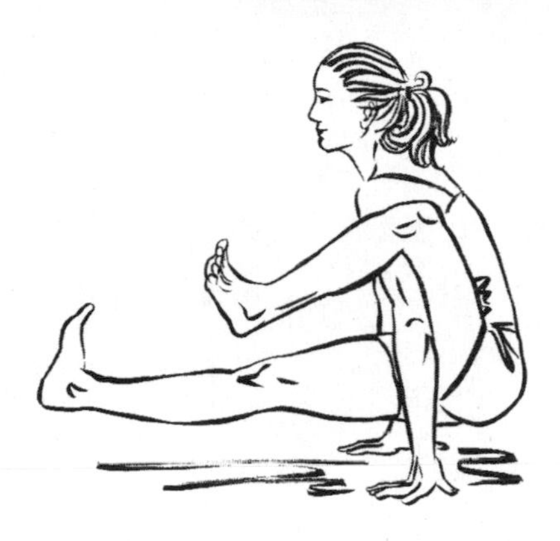

1. In Baby Cradle Pose, holding on to your right ankle, lift your right leg over your arm pulling it up as high as possible on your arm. Clamp the leg as you slide your hands to the sides of your hips. Extend your opposite leg forward. (Try setting your hands on blocks if you're having trouble.)
2. Align with the bigger flow, and draw from your fingers into your heart. Engage your legs; draw from your toes inward and hug your legs in toward each other.
3. Slide your hips back and lift your buttocks and legs off the floor.
4. Celebrate your uniqueness by offering back out from your heart and rooting your hands into the earth. Shine out fully for a few breaths before trying the other side.

Chapter 7

Charging Your Core: Abdominals

Working your abdominals is perhaps the most difficult and the most gratifying exercise. Your effort is well worth it, though, as abdominal work increases energy, aids in digestion, and helps strengthen your lower back.

In the energetic system of the *chakras*, the abdominal area, or third chakra, rules over your power. In Sanskrit, the third chakra, in your abdomen, is named the "lustrous gem" and is the color of the sun. As you work your abdomen, you charge your core as the sun charges the earth. You will soon notice that abdominal work kindles your internal *agni*, energizing your body and stimulating digestive fire.

It's important to practice hip-opening poses before abdominals so your legs and groin are stretched. That way, the front of your groin doesn't tighten.

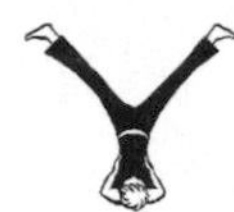

Yoga Speak

Part of the energetic science of yoga, a **chakra** is one of seven major centers where energy is received, processed, and transmitted throughout your body. The word literally means "wheel" or "disc." **Agni,** or fire, can refer to the heat within the body that increases circulation and secretions.

Let's go through all the alignment steps as they apply to abdominal asanas:

1. Begin by receiving your breath, letting it expand you from the inside out.
2. To use your abdominals and not your back, emphasize drawing from your legs in toward your hips, plugging into the core of your pelvis.
3. Turn your thighs slightly in toward each other and then back and apart in Inner Spiral.
4. Keeping the top of your thighs back, scoop your tailbone in.
5. Then, as much as you are drawing in, extend out to maintain balance.

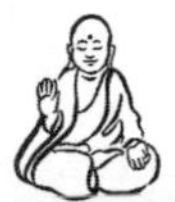

Be Mindful

If you have difficulties with your lower back, be careful working with abdominals. Be sure you're using your abdominal muscles and not your back muscles, as the later can cause strain. Proceed slowly until you strengthen your core. Try bending your knees and holding the postures for short periods of time. If you feel pain or strain, bend your knees and release immediately.

Boat/Navasana

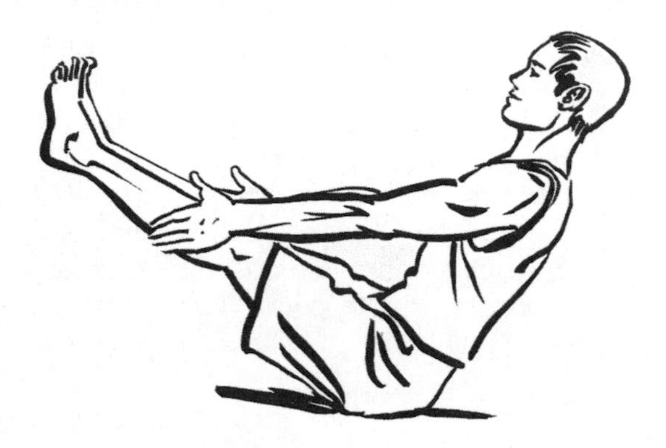

1. Sitting up tall, draw your knees into your chest.
2. As you hold on to the back of your thighs, find your balance point by rolling back onto your tailbone.
3. Stretching your arms forward, straighten your legs. Try to keep your head and feet the same height as you lengthen your spine.
4. As you inhale, embrace your power by drawing in from your fingers and flexed feet into your body. As you exhale, extend that power out, shining out as bright as the sun.
5. Hold for as many breaths as you can until your muscles tire, up to one minute.

Half Boat/Ardha Navasana

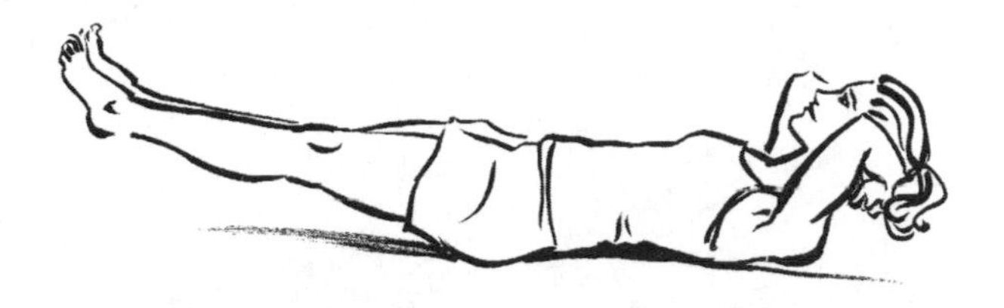

1. Lying on your back on the floor, interlace your fingers, placing your heads behind your head.
2. Draw your knees into your chest.
3. As you lift your head and heart, extend your legs straight. Your head and legs should be at a 30-degree angle from the floor. You can press your head into your hands to support your neck.
4. Try holding for at least five breaths to one minute.

Leg Lifts

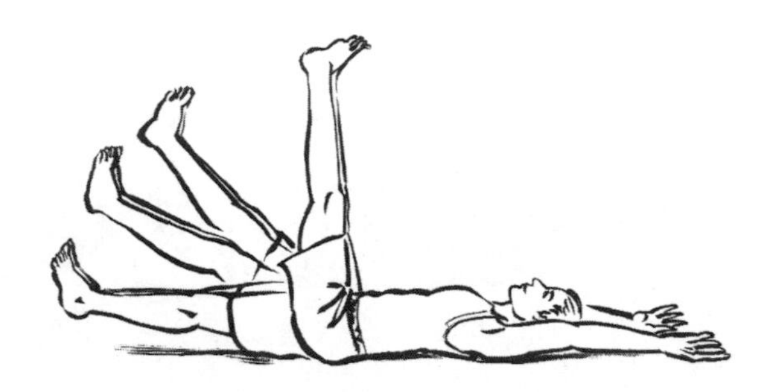

1. Lay on your back, "standing" in Mountain Pose.
2. Bring your arms overhead as you lift your legs up to the ceiling.
3. As the sun charges its core, charge your core, drawing from your feet into your pelvis.
4. Without losing this charge, extend from your pelvis back out through your feet like rays of the sun.
5. Slowly lower your legs 30 degrees and pause for a few breaths.
6. Lower your legs 30 degrees more and pause.
7. Now lower your legs an inch off the floor and pause. Are you breathing? Keep scooping your tailbone, using your abdominal muscles and not your back. Try it again.

Turning Round the Belly/ Jathara Parivartanasana

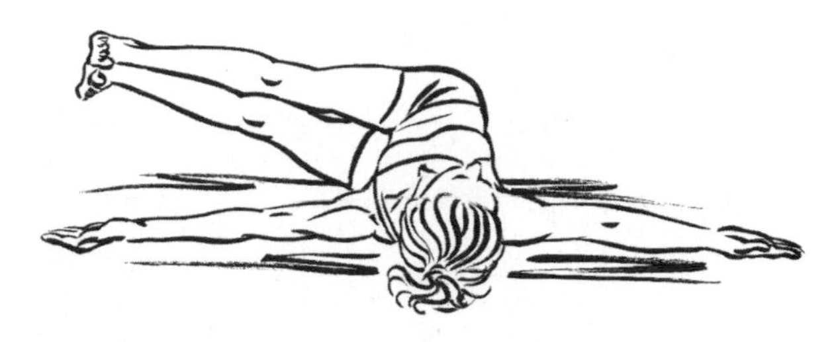

1. Begin on your back, placing your arms in T position, extending them out perpendicular to your body.
2. Bend your knees and swing your hips to the left so your legs and buttocks move to the left side of your mat.
3. Extend your legs, and slowly, with your exhalation, lower them to your right an inch off the floor.
4. Align with your innate strength, drawing from your feet into your pelvis. Celebrate this power by extending from your pelvis back out through your feet and spreading your toes.
5. Pause for a few breathes and then slowly lift your legs back up to center.
6. Swing your hips to the right and then lower your legs to the left.
7. Repeat a couple times on each side.

Turning Your World Upside Down: Inversions

Inversions are tremendously nourishing and detoxifying to the body. All your body's systems are positively affected by inversions: by reversing the flow of blood, the head and upper body receive more blood and the lymph system drains. After coming out of an inversion, the circulatory system is renewed with fresh energy and the body is recharged. When you invert, your organs get to hang, reducing the effects of gravity and revitalizing your organs and glands. The endocrine glands that regulate your immune system are also strengthened.

As you invert, you literally turn your world upside down. This gives you a different vision, or perspective, of the world and yourself in it. Inversions also sooth the nervous system, helping you become more internalized.

With so many positive effects, it's not hard to see why inversions are emphasized in yoga. In fact, Headstand/Sirsasana is dubbed "the king of all yoga poses" and Shoulderstand/Sarvangasana, "the queen." These asanas are so beneficial because they are radically different from anything you do during the course of your day.

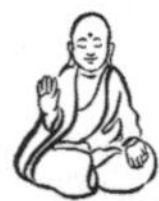

Be Mindful

Inversions can be really scary for the beginner and even for more experienced practitioners. One of the greatest fears in inverted poses is falling over backward, into the "unknown." For beginners, practicing next to the wall is essential. It provides support so you can find your balance.

Because so many of your "buttons" will be pushed when practicing inversions, these poses are incredibly gratifying to achieve.

Pose Prep

Each pose in this chapter is broken into two poses: the preparatory pose and the full pose. Beginners might want to work just with the prep pose until you feel more steady and confident.

For the prep poses, you might need a *block* and *strap*. For full Shoulderstand, you need blankets. There are also many contraindications for (reasons you shouldn't do) inversions (see the following "Be Mindful" section). This also provides alternatives for those who find they are not medically able to practice inversions.

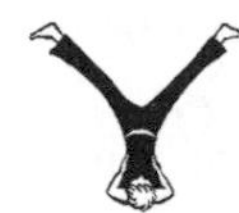

Yoga Speak

Blocks, straps, and blankets are some of the props used in yoga. A **strap** is used to hold arms or legs in place or as an extension of the arms. Cotton yoga straps have a buckle and are 6 to 10 feet long. *Sticky mats,* the most popular prop, are a type of yoga mat that is slightly sticky and helps you to not slip in your poses.

Before turning everything upside down, here are a few important points to focus on with inversions:

The most important part of alignment in inversions is a strong foundation. Just as a house built on a cracked foundation will falter, so will you if your foundation is not centered and steady.

Remember to stay engaged. Use muscular energy, particularly in your legs, which tend to become passive.

Keep your shoulder blades firmly on your back. If you round your shoulders forward, you can strain your neck, shoulders, or arms.

Practice the following alignment standing in Mountain Pose: place a hand behind your head, and press your head back into your hand. Now your neck should be in line with your spine, the base of your skull over your tailbone. As you inhale, feel your whole chest expanding. Keeping this expansiveness, especially in the sides of your ribs, draw your shoulder blades onto your back. Your shoulder blades stay on your back, the top of your arm bones stay up as your shoulder blades softly relax down. Your heart stays lifted.

The soft palate is the Focal Point for Headstand and Shoulderstand. For Peacock Feather, it is the heart.

Don't forget to breathe!

Transition is very important for inversions. It's good to slowly release into Child's Pose, keeping your head down to prevent dizziness. Once in Child's Pose, take a few breaths before slowly coming up.

Inversion Cautions

Inversions are not recommended if you have unmedicated high or low blood pressure, a detached retina, or are menstruating. If you have neck or shoulder issues, modifications can be made to strengthen these areas. Check with your doctor to see if it's okay to perform inversions and then work with a certified yoga teacher to ensure proper alignment. Inversions are also not recommended if you are pregnant and have not been regularly practicing these poses.

Why no inversions during menstruation? Different schools of yoga have varied opinions on yoga and menstruation. Some schools believe no inversions should be done during menstruating, while others suggest avoiding them the first 3 days or when the menses is strong; other schools think a woman's whole practice should be limited during this time. Remember, yoga was originally created by men for men, so the effects of yoga and menstruation on the body have not been studied for very long. When you are menstruating, blood and energy are flowing downward. Inversions reverse the flow of blood and energy. Therefore, inversions may confuse the body, resulting in a temporary cessation of menstrual flow, later causing increased flow and cramping. Each body and each period is different. Listen to your body and its needs, and experiment with what works for you.

If you have any of these considerations, don't skip this chapter! If you're injured, there's a safe inversion for you (Restorative Legs Against the Wall). For those menstruating, there's a restorative pose for you (Supine Bound Angle).

Headstand Prep/Sirsasana Prep

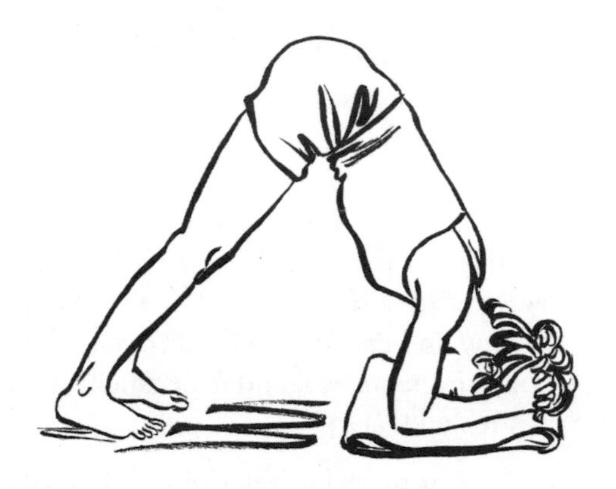

1. Fold your sticky mat in half, and place it two inches from a clear wall.
2. Place your forearms down on the mat so your elbows are shoulder-width apart. With your hands one hand's width away from the wall, interlace your fingers. Your hands should stay rigid; do not let them drop over. Press your forearms, wrists, and the outer edges of the hands down into the earth.
3. Place your head in between your hands so your hands cradle your head. Align with your courage, drawing your shoulder blades firmly onto the back of your heart.
4. Curling your toes under, straighten your legs, extending your hips up to the ceiling. You should now be on the crown of your head. If you tend to have a flat neck (head protrudes forward) be ½ inch closer to your forehead.

5. Keep rooting your arms, wrist, hands, and even your head down as you extend your hips up.
6. Hold for a few breaths and then release into Child's Pose.

Headstand/Sirsasana

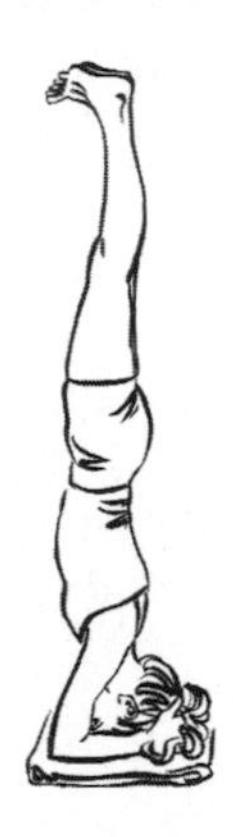

1. Come into Headstand Prep.
2. Walk your feet in toward your head until you cannot walk in any more.
3. Be sure your shoulder blades are still flat on your back and that your back is not rounding. (If you have tight shoulders, you may want to stay in the prep.)
4. *For beginners:* Extend one leg straight up toward the ceiling; the other leg will lift and follow. You may have to slightly kick up the first few times. Keep your kicking leg straight. *For experienced:* Bring up both legs together.
5. If you're practicing against the wall, bend one knee and place that foot against the wall while stretching your other leg up to the sky. Scoop your tailbone, drawing it up to the ceiling. Most people overarch their back when upside down; scooping your tailbone eliminates that.

6. Feed yourself confidence, drawing from your elbows and legs into your palate, creating integration. Strengthen your foundation, rooting your head, wrists, and hands down as you extend your legs up, dragging your heels up the wall. Remember to breathe evenly.
7. When you feel your muscles getting tired, release into Child's Pose. (For beginners, keep one leg bent with the foot pressing into the wall as you lower your straight leg first. Your bent leg can slowly follow. This way you can come down with ease.)

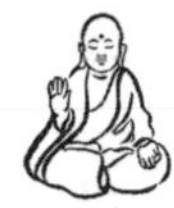

Be Mindful

Make sure that your shoulderblades are engaged, moving up and onto your back. If your back is rounded (shoulders not flat on your back), you can compress your cervical (neck) vertebrae. When done correctly, Headstand actually lengthens the cervical spine.

Peacock Feather Prep/ Pinca Mayurasana Prep

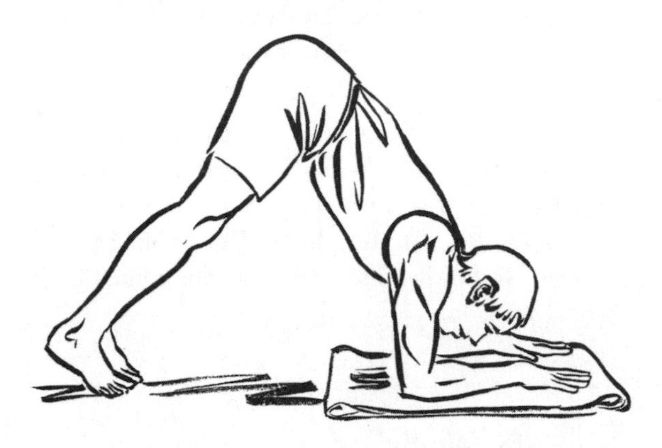

1. Come onto all fours, facing an empty wall. Bring your hands one hand width away from the wall.
2. As you inhale, feel your whole body swelling from the inside out. Embrace your strength, and isometrically swipe your hands into each other. Draw from your fingers energetically into your heart so your shoulder blades come flat on your back.
3. Keeping your body's fullness, as you exhale, allow your heart to melt with offering and extend from your heart through your hands, rooting the four corners of each hand.
4. Keeping your shoulder blades flat on your back and your inner body expansive, slowly lower your forearms to the floor. Move slowly and with awareness to maintain alignment. When your

elbows are on the floor, they should be shoulder-width apart. If your elbows are wider, try again, as your shoulder blades came off your back.

5. Curling your toes under, slowly extend your legs, reaching your hips up toward the sky. Your head should not be on the floor. Look at your hands.
6. Maintain your commitment to a strong foundation, rooting the arms down. Hold for a few breaths.

Repeating this exercise a few times strengthens the rhomboid muscles responsible for drawing the shoulder blades onto the back.

Peacock Feather/Pinca Mayurasana

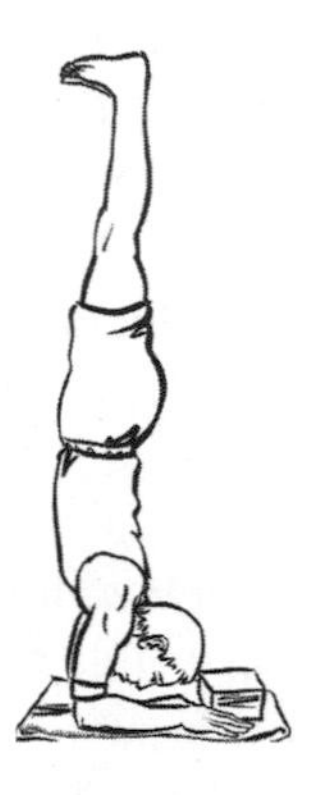

Beginners need a block and a strap.

1. Make a strap shoulder-width apart, and place it on your upper arms just above your elbows. This prevents your elbows from splaying apart and thus helps maintain your shoulder blades flat on your back.
2. Place the block's long side against the wall, with your hands around the lower corners of the block. If you make an L shape with your thumb and index finger, you can link them around the block.
3. Come into Peacock Feather Prep.
4. Walk your feet into your hands until you cannot walk in any more.
5. Take in a deep breath and open to something bigger. As you exhale, be sure your heart is still melted and your back is long and not rounding.

6. When you're sure your shoulder blades are flat on your back, gently kick one leg up at a time.
7. The lower back tends to overarch; to remedy this, bend one leg and place the foot against the wall. With the other leg straight, scoop your tailbone and extend it up to the sky. Straighten your other leg. Look down at your hands.
8. Be strength and stability as you root your forearms and hands down as you drag your heels up the wall, extending in both directions.
9. Playfully melt your heart without overarching your back.
10. Hold for a few breaths up to a few minutes, depending on your strength, and then release one leg at a time.

Shoulderstand Prep/ Sarvangasana Prep

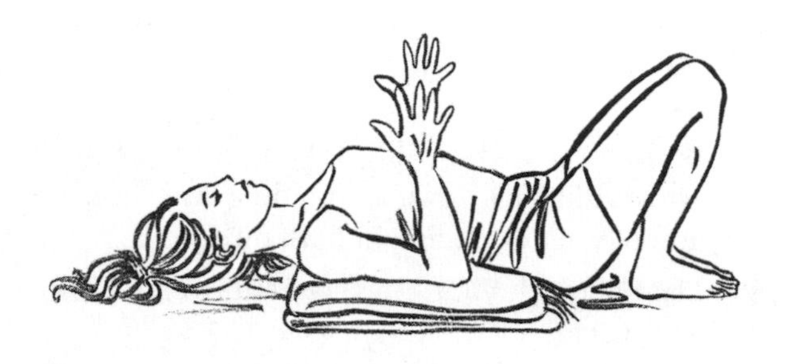

You need at least two blankets.

1. Fold your sticky mat in half. Stack your blankets one on top of the other so you have at least 2 inches of thickness. The top line of the blankets should be neat. Place your blankets on the top edge of your folded mat and then fold over the rest of the mat. The mat should cover about ⅔ of the blankets with the top third open.
2. Lie on your blankets so your shoulders are on the blankets and your neck is off. There should be a few inches of space between the curve of your neck and the floor. Leave a ½ inch of blanket above your shoulders, for as you roll back, your shoulders will also roll back and you want to keep them on the blankets.

3. Bend your elbows so your palms face each other and press your upper arms into the blankets. You'll feel your shoulder blades curl onto your back and your heart lifting and expanding. Now you are ready for the full pose.

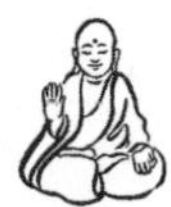

Be Mindful

Keeping the back of your neck long (chin doesn't lift), press the back of your skull into the floor. This exercise strengthens the back of your neck, releasing tension in the neck and shoulders.

Shoulderstand/Sarvangasana

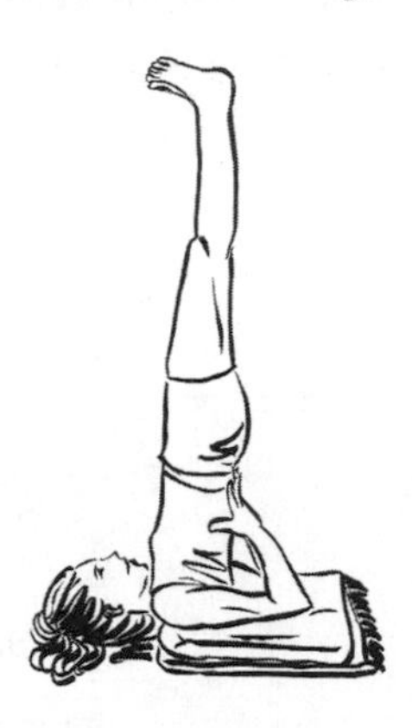

1. Come into Shoulderstand Prep. Release your arms at your sides. Roll your knees into your chest, lifting your buttocks away from the floor. (At first you may need to rock from a seated position and swing back and up.)
2. Place your hands on your back, the closer to your shoulder blades the more support you have. For stability, cross your legs and hug your thighs in as you walk your elbows together (you want them shoulder-width apart) and your hands closer to your shoulders. Once you have adjusted, uncross your legs.
3. Feed your innate strength; draw energetically from your elbows to your palate, lifting your heart. Your chin should be slightly tucked in to your chest. Engage your legs. Reaffirm your stability, and root your arms and shoulders and head (keeping the back of your neck long) down as you extend out through your legs.

4. Try increasing your holding each time you practice this pose, working up to a few minutes.
5. To release, follow Plow Pose.

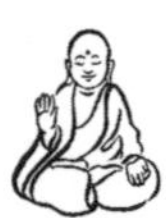

Be Mindful

Make sure your shoulders stay on the blanket. If they roll off, you'll feel unsteady. If you have difficulty coming into the pose, try setting up your blankets and mat a few feet away from a wall. You can walk up the wall to come into the pose.

Plow/Halasana

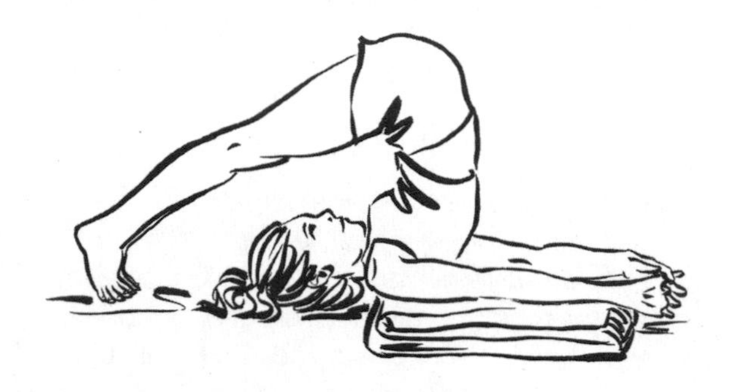

1. From Shoulderstand, draw your feet over your head toward the floor. If you can't touch the floor, try "walking" down a wall.
2. Align with your power, feeding the core of your pose. Draw from your fingers and feet into your palate. From your soft palate, press your feet into the wall or toes into the floor, extending out through your heels.
3. Interlace your fingers behind your back. Roll your shoulder blades more onto your back. (You can roll onto one shoulder and pull the opposite blade under and then do the other side.)
4. Lift and expand your heart, radiating your heart's desire. Extend your hips up to the sky. Hold for a few breaths or one minute.
5. Open your hands apart to prepare for releasing the pose. You can hold onto the sides of your blankets for stability. Slowly roll back down, dropping your buttocks back onto the floor.

Supine Easy Pose/ Supta Baddha Sukhasana

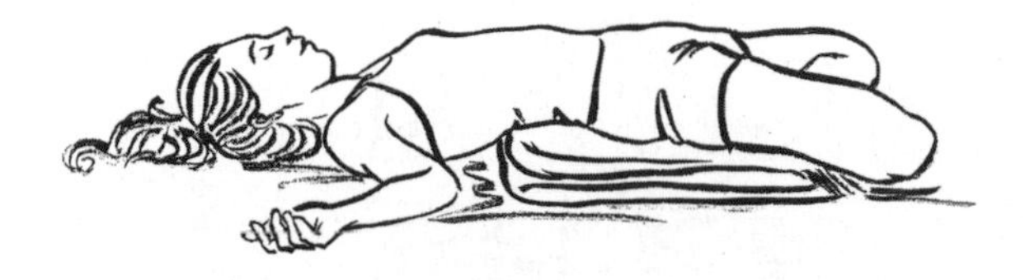

This asana is great after Shoulderstand and Plow because it passively opens your chest.

1. After you release Plow, stay lying down and slide yourself back so your hips are on the blankets. Both shoulder blades should be on the floor, your arms should be out to a T position, and your chest is open.
2. Bending your knees, cross your ankles and let your knees drop open so the sides of your legs are resting on the floor. Legs are in Simple Seated Pose/Sukhasana.
3. After a few breaths, reverse the crossing of your legs and relax for the same amount of time.
4. To release, draw your knees into your chest and roll over onto one side. After a few breaths, press up to a seated position.

Restorative Legs Against the Wall/ Viparini Karani

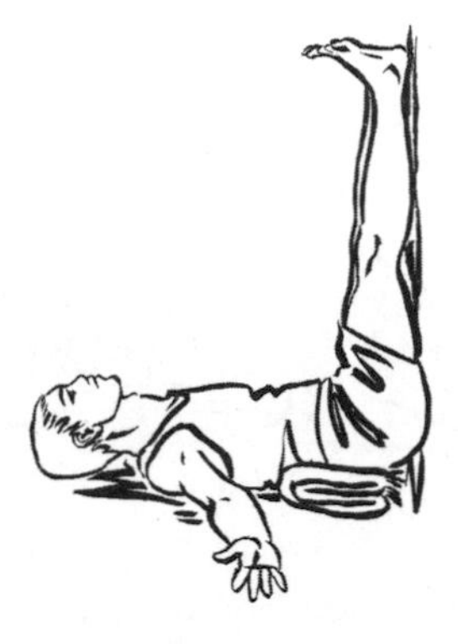

If you're unable to do other inversions due to injuries, this is a great and gentle alternative inversion. You need two blankets and a wall.

1. Fold your two blankets so they're approximately 1 foot wide and 3 or 4 inches thick. Place the long side of the blankets 2 or 3 inches away from the wall.
2. Sit on the blanket with one hip against the wall. One buttock check should be on the blanket while the one close to the wall is hanging off.
3. Pivot your hips toward the wall as you lie back and extend your legs up the wall. Your hips and lower back should be on the blanket; your buttocks should be slightly hanging off the blanket.
4. Actively flex your feet.
5. Hold for 2 to 10 minutes. To release, bend your knees and roll over onto your side for a few breaths.

Menstrual Pose: Supine Bound Angle/Supta Baddha Konasana

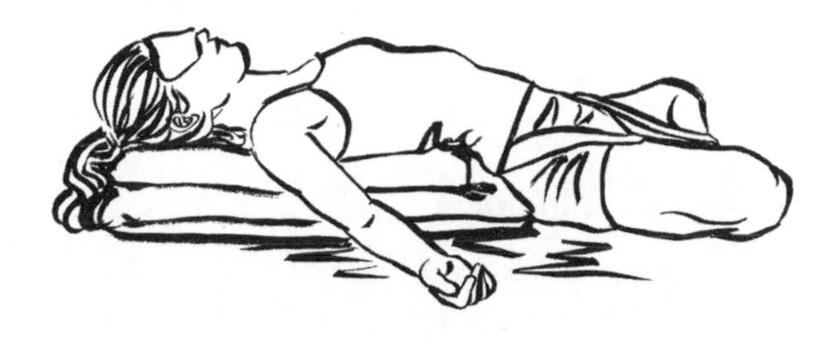

You will need a blanket, mat, and strap. If you're menstruating, you can replace inversions with this pose. It reduces menstrual cramping.

1. Roll your sticky mat up or fold a blanket into thirds so it's as long as your mat.
2. Sit against the mat your buttocks on the floor.
3. Bring the soles of your feet together, knees wide apart.
4. Make a giant loop with your strap, place it over your head, and slide it around your torso. The loop should be on your lower back.
5. Take the other end of your strap under your feet. The strap is now over your legs. Adjust the strap so your legs feel supported. You may need blankets under your thighs for extra support.

6. Lie back on your mat, and enjoy the gift of your breath. Relax in this pose for a couple minutes or longer.
7. To transition out of the pose, bring your knees together so you can slide your feet out of the strap and roll over onto one side for a few breaths.

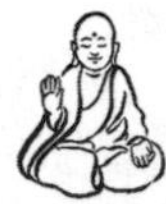

Be Mindful

This pose is excellent for relieving menstrual cramps, especially when combined with forward bends. Try this sequence: after releasing this pose, hold a forward bend for one minute. Then lay back on your blankets with your legs extended for one minute. Finally, repeat with another forward bend. (Please see Chapter 11 for Forward Bend

Chapter 9

Opening Your Heart: Backbends

Invigorating and energizing, backbends cultivate a sense of courage and are natural anti-depressants. Backbends radically open the chest, allowing the lungs to swell with fresh oxygen. For this reason, backbends are excellent poses to practice for those with breathing difficulties such as asthma.

Backbends also physically and energetically open the heart, which for most people tends to be quite armored. Courage develops as you shed layers of protection and you open your heart to receive the pulsation of life. When you open your heart in this way, a sense of enthusiasm, vitality, and strength follow.

A balance between flexibility and strength is necessary in achieving stability with backbends. All the categories of asanas you have done in the previous chapters have prepared you for these poses. Moving into back-body (a part of you that you cannot see) is an exploration of the unknown. Bring your adventurous spirit along as you practice these asanas.

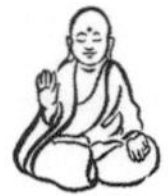

Be Mindful

Backbending requires open hips and shoulders. It's important to do some standing poses, hip openers, and quad stretches before practicing backbends.

Backbend Fundamentals

In this chapter, you will find several poses ideal for beginners and for those with tighter hips and shoulders, including Cobra Variation, Half Bow, Full Bow, and Bridge poses. There are also more challenging postures, such as Upward Facing Dog, Bridge with One Leg Extended, Upward Facing Bow, and Camel poses. Please respect your body and work with those asanas you have already practiced with your teacher.

Here are some important points of alignment to emphasize in backbends:

- You need a strong foundation. Your feet should be parallel and steadfast. Your hips and shoulders should be even and on the same plane.
- To align your hips and lower back, you must emphasize Inner Spiral before subtly scooping your tailbone (Outer Spiral). If you're performing this correctly, you should have no lower back discomfort.

- Try to bend more from the back of your heart than from your lower back. The lower back tends to be hyper-mobile and, therefore, less stable. The back of the heart tends to be stuck.
- Remember to open to receive your breath. The sides of your ribs need to be long. Your body needs to lengthen rather than shorten.
- Shoulder and neck alignment: The sides of your ribs lengthen as they swell with Prana. Your neck is not protruding forward, but the base of your skull is over your tailbone. Your shoulder blades are flat on your back. The top of your arm bone stays up, and your heart stays lifted as your shoulder blades relax down and your ribs soften.

Backbend Cautions

Backbends should not create a pulling sensation or discomfort in your back or any other area of your body.

Although correctly aligned backbends can be helpful for some back conditions, it's important to check with your teacher and doctor before working in backbends. When doing poses lying on your back, try placing a block in between your feet to relieve any mild back discomfort. (Use the block in whatever way is closest to inner hip-width apart.) Bringing your big toes against the block provides a reference point to see if your toes turn out when you come up into a backbend. Turning the toes out is a common habit that compresses the lower back. Emphasize Inner Spiral, making sure you're not putting more weight on the outer edges of your feet. Try opening your upper back more and your lower back less.

Upward Facing Bow, Upward Facing Dog, and Camel poses require strong and integrated back muscles, arms, and shoulders. If you have injuries in any of these areas, please work with your teacher to modify these poses for you. Your shoulder blades must be firmly on your back to stay integrated.

If you have knee difficulties, please be mindful of your foot and leg alignment. Concentrate on isometrically swiping your feet (without moving them) in toward each other so your shins hug in. As you keep your shins hugging in, widen the back of your thighs with Inner Spiral. You can also try placing a sock behind each knee so there's no compression.

If you're pregnant, your body is in a natural backbend that deepens as your pregnancy advances, and there's little need for you to practice backbends. If you do practice these asanas, do mini-backbends. Do not rest your back flat on the floor after your first trimester.

Cobra Variation/ Bhujangasana Variation

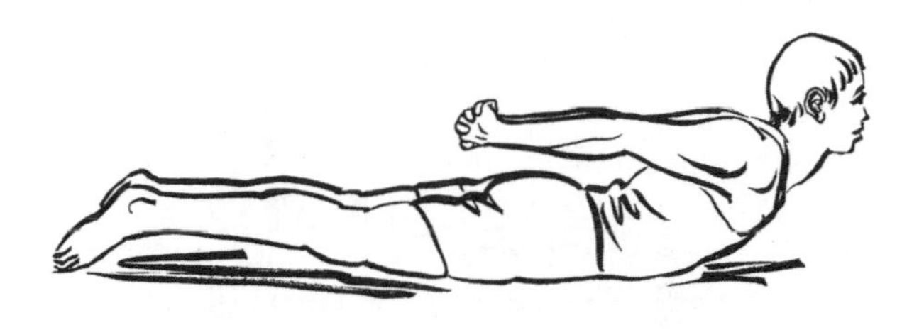

1. Lie face down on the floor. Align with your power, hugging your shins in and down, scooping your tailbone toward your toes to engage your legs.
2. Interlace your fingers behind you. If you have tight shoulders and cannot reach your hands, try holding onto a strap with each hand. Place your hands as close together as possible on the strap.
3. As you inhale, root your pelvis down and lift your chest. Feed the pose by drawing from your toes into your pelvis and then extending from the pelvis back out from the toes.
4. Celebrate the gift of life, your heart shining out. To enhance this celebration, you can also draw energetically from your fingers into your heart balancing the action by extending out through your fingers and heart. Hold for a few breaths.
5. Can you melt your heart without losing the lift in your chest?

Upward Facing Dog/ Urdhva Mukha Svanasana

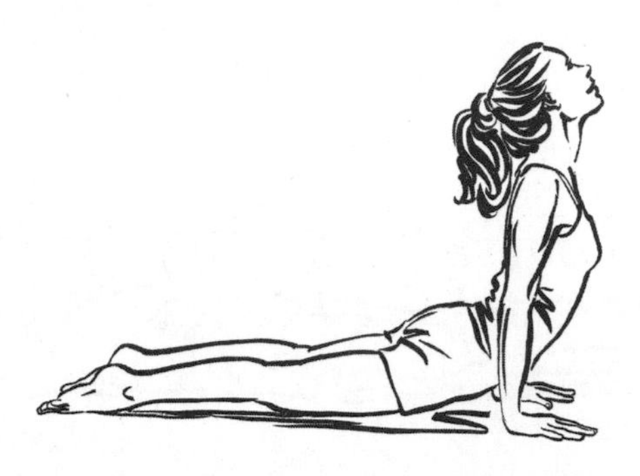

The difference between Up Dog and full Cobra is that in Up Dog your pelvis is off the floor. This is a more advanced asana, so you may want to stay with Cobra, especially if you have back issues.

1. Lying on your belly, slide your hands under your shoulders. Engage your legs as you lift your chest up into Cobra (see Chapter 3).
2. As you inhale, feel your sides lengthening as you receive your fullness and move the back of your ears backward so your neck is aligned with your spine. Draw your shoulder blades onto your back as you joyfully lift and expand your heart.
3. Claw the floor as you expand your chest forward through your hands while your pelvis slides forward, lifting away slightly from the floor.
4. Keeping your heart lifted, relax your shoulder blades down. If your elbows are slightly bent, it'll be easier to keep your shoulder blades back.

Half Bow/Ardha Dhanurasana

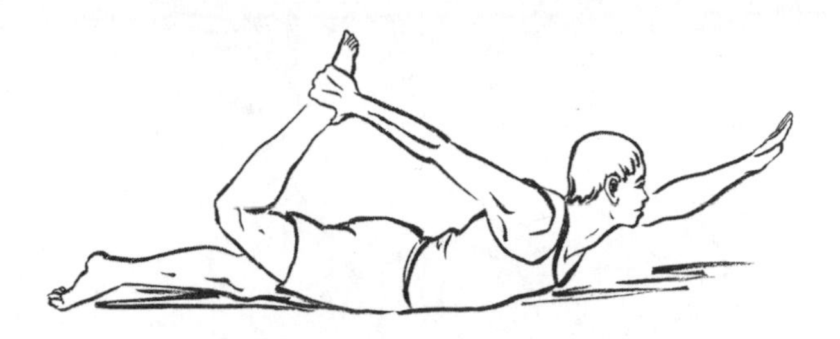

1. Begin by lying face down on the floor. Bend your right knee and grasp your right foot with your right hand. If you can't reach, try holding a strap looped around your foot.
2. Extend your left arm out above your head, along the floor. Scoop your tailbone toward your toes. Kick your right leg back as you lift your head, chest, and left arm.
3. Balance engaging with extending out, and stay equally weighted on both hips.
4. With your next inhalation, you receive Prana, the energy that feeds all things, and your chest swells and rises with that nourishment. Enhance this pulsation by offering back out your unique creativity and expanding your heart.
5. As you exhale, maintain your fullness as your skin softens.
6. Hold for a few breaths up to one minute, and then repeat on the opposite side.

Bow/Dhanurasana

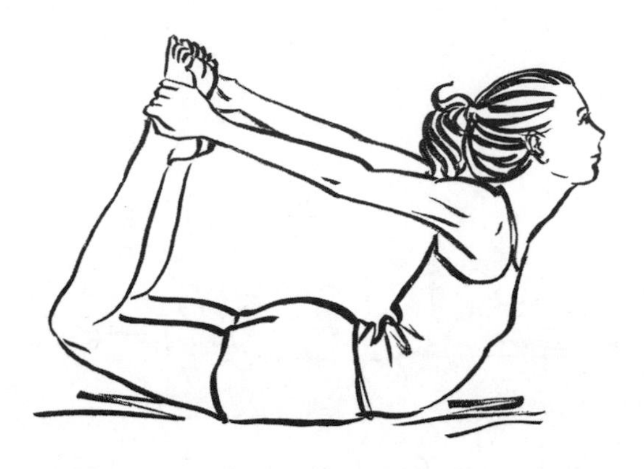

1. Lie face down on the floor. Scoop your tailbone, and bend both knees grasping, onto both feet. If you can't reach with one or both hands, use a strap around both ankles.
2. As you inhale, with an adventurous spirit, draw your legs up and back, lifting your chest up. The more you kick up and back, the more your chest will rise and your full heart can soften.
3. Be sure your neck is in line with your spine.
4. Repeat this one or two more times, seeing if you can relax into the effort more. Can you breathe fully?

Bridge/Setubhandha Sarvangasana

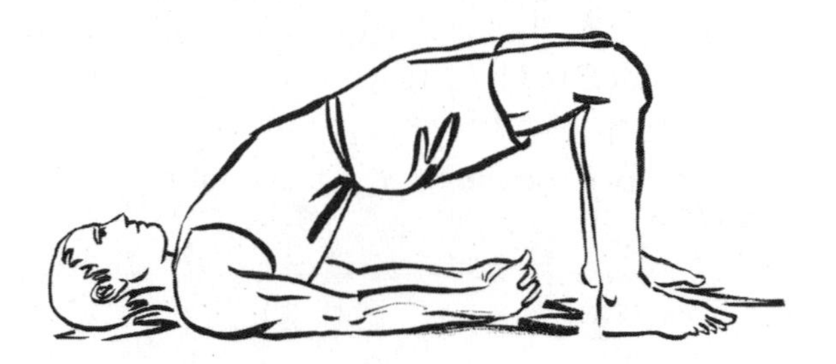

1. Lie on your back, with your knees bent and your feet inner hip-width apart and parallel. Your ankles should be under your knees. As you line up physically, align with your intention. Enjoy the fullness of your breath.
2. Without moving them, draw your feet energetically into each other and into your body. You will feel your strong legs engaging and your pelvis wanting to rise.
3. Turn your thighs slightly in toward each other and down toward the floor (Inner Spiral). You will feel your buttocks press into the floor and your lower back arch.
4. Gently scoop your tailbone as you lift your pelvis toward the sky.
5. Roll your arms and shoulders under you, and interlace your fingers.

6. Feed your pose by drawing from your feet and fingers into the soft palate. Offer back just as much as you are receiving by extending from the palate out through your heart and knees, lengthening in two opposite directions. Be sure your chin is not lifted but is slightly tucked into your chest so the back of your neck remains long.
7. Are the four corners of your feet evenly weighted?

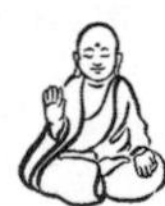

Be Mindful

Lower back pain in backbends is often caused by turning the toes out so you loose Inner Spiral. Because you can't see your feet, it might be difficult to tell if you are turning out. Try placing a block between your feet so your toes have a reference point to press into.

Bridge with One Leg Extended/ Eka Pada Setubhandha Sarvangasana

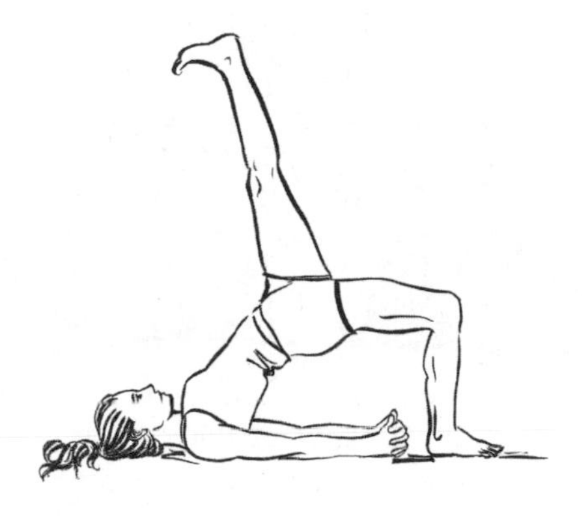

1. From Bridge, press your right foot evenly into the floor, hugging your right shin into your left.
2. As you inhale, draw your left knee into your chest, and exhaling with celebration, extend your leg, trying to "stand" on the ceiling.
3. The tendency is for the right leg to bow out, so keep enhancing self-support by pressing your inner foot down as you hug your shin in.
4. Press your arms and shoulders into the floor as you lift and your expansive heart shines.
5. Release your left foot and lift your other leg.

Upward Facing Bow Prep/ Urdhva Dhanurasana Prep

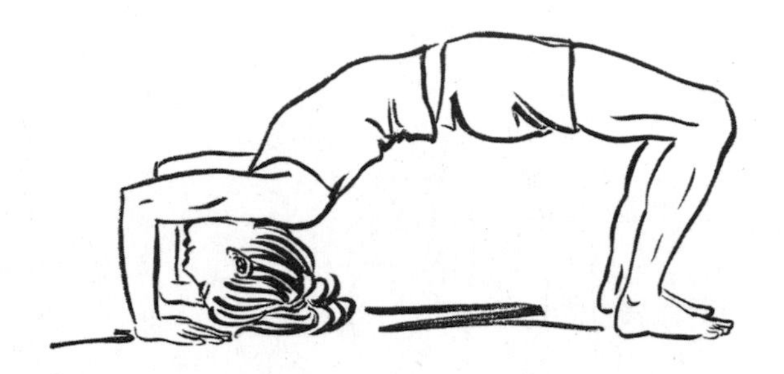

1. Lying on your back, place your hands on the floor alongside your ears. Your fingers should be pointing in toward your shoulders.
2. Place your feet on the floor hip-width apart and parallel so your ankles are under your knees.
3. Draw energetically from your elbows in toward your armpits so your shoulder blades come flat onto your back.
4. Gently turn your thighs in toward each other and down toward the floor and then subtly scoop your tailbone. Lift your pelvis up into Bridge Pose.
5. Pressing your hands into the earth, see if you can lift onto the top of your head.
6. Again, align with your true nature, draw energetically from your elbows into your armpits so your shoulder blades come flat on your back and your heart opens.

7. If you are on your head, you're ready to try the full pose.

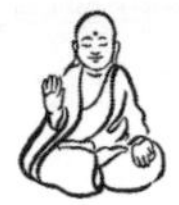

Be Mindful

If you can't lift onto your head, try using baseboard trim on a wall an inch or two from the floor. With your fingertips on the floor, rest the base of your palm on the trim. The angle will help those with tight shoulders or weak wrists.

Upward Facing Bow/ Urdhva Dhanurasana

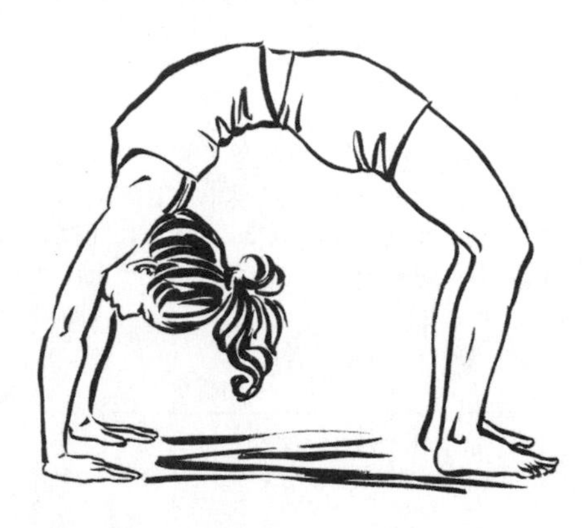

1. From Upward Facing Dog Prep, draw from your elbows into your heart so your shoulder blades are magnetized onto your back. Pressing your hands into the floor, fully extend your arms, lifting your head off the floor.
2. Look down at your hands. Channel your power, isometrically swiping your hands into each other. Work your feet in the same way. Keep rooting your hands and feet into the supportive earth.
3. How much do you want to align with your fullness? That is how much you hug in. As you inhale, feed the core of the pose, drawing your hands and feet energetically into your heart. Receive the pulsation of life flowing through you.
4. As you exhale, lift and expand your heart, celebrating this gift.
5. Take a few breaths and release. Repeat at least once or twice more.

Camel Prep/Ustrasana Prep

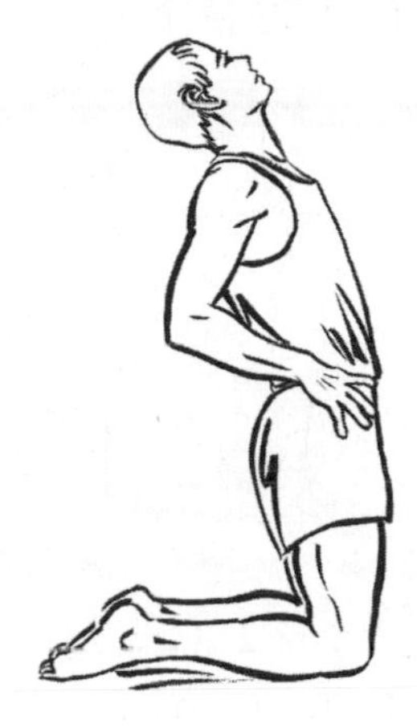

1. Kneel with your knees inner hip-width apart. If you're not a deep back bender, curl your toes under or place blocks on either side of your outer heels.
2. As you inhale, feel your whole chest lifting and expanding.
3. Place a hand behind your head, and press your head back into that hand. Your neck will move back in line with your spine. Draw your shoulder blades onto the back of your heart as your heart keeps lifting.
4. Turn your inner thighs slightly in toward each other, and move the top of your thighs back, widening the back of your pelvis, and then gently scoop your tailbone.
5. Now you are ready for the full pose.

Camel/Ustrasana

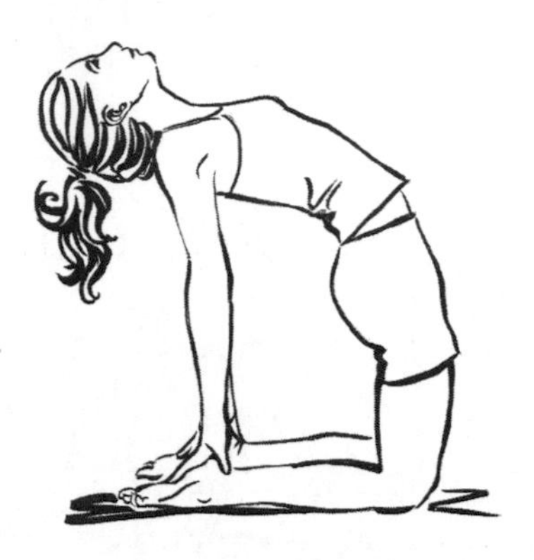

1. From Camel Prep, as you inhale, receive your fullness. We are all bigger and brighter than we visualize ourselves. With your expansive heart open, look up.
2. As you exhale, place one hand at a time on your heels (or blocks), trusting yourself that you will find them. (Try not to look!)
3. If your neck is aligned properly, you can release your head back.
4. Stay with your breath as you inhale, feeling your brightness expanding, and as you exhale, softening your skin and your ribs.
5. Hold for a minimum of a few breaths. Try Camel once more.

Chapter 10

Wringing Out Your Tension: Spinal Twists

Twists are an excellent way to release tension from the body. As you twist, your body is wrung free of toxins, as a washcloth is wrung free of dirty water. When you release, fresh blood pours back into the area, nourishing it. As you twist, you gently squeeze your abdominal area and kidneys, helping regulate digestion and elimination. Glands, organs, and your circulatory system are cleansed and refreshed.

Twists are wonderful for the back and spine and are an ideal exercise for back discomfort. Twists enhance the circulation in your entire spine. Try a twist the next time your back feels stiff. If your back feels tweaky after a backbend, do a gentle twist rather than a forward bend.

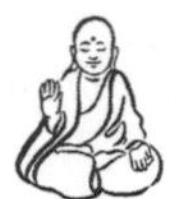

Be Mindful

A twist is not a rotation. People tend to move their bodies as one unit. A twist differentiates itself by keeping one area stable as another area moves. For example, if you do a twist in your office chair, your hips stay facing forward as your chest rotates to allow your arms to hold on to the back of the chair.

There are a few points of alignment to keep in mind for twists:

- Remember to breathe.
- Hug into your center and create resistance.
- Keep your foundation steady.
- As you inhale, lengthen your spine; as you exhale, twist.
- Let the twist be initiated from the opposite and back side of your body (direction you are turning away from).
- Try to keep an inner spaciousness on the side you're twisting.

Twist Cautions

Be respectful to your body and do not force yourself deeper into a twist than you can comfortably go. Allow your breath to move you more fully in the asana.

As in seated poses, if your lower back collapses backward, you'll need to sit on a blanket to support your lower back.

If you're pregnant, check with your doctor to learn if twisting is okay. For most pregnancies, adjusting the direction of the seated twists so the belly is not pressing against any other part of the body is an acceptable modification. After the first trimester, you should not lie on your back.

Knees to the Side

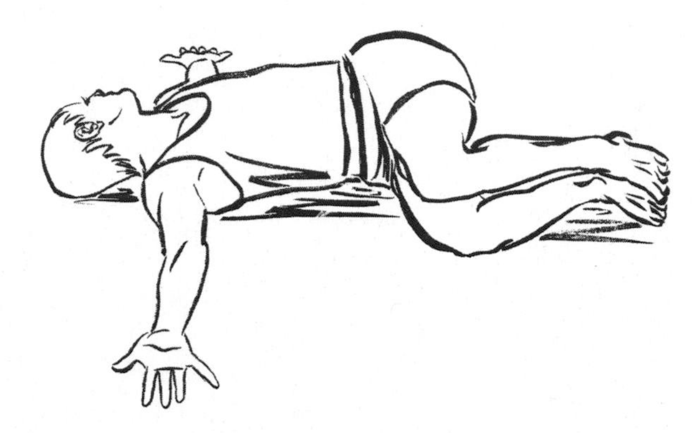

1. Lie on your back with your arms out in T position, palms facing up.
2. Open to receive the pulsation of your breath. As you inhale, draw your knees into your chest. (If you have sciatica, place a blanket between your knees.)
3. As you exhale, drop your knees to the right. Be sure your left shoulder blade is on the floor. If it's not, back off from the twist until it is. (This strengthens the rotator cuff muscles.)
4. Turn your head to the left.
5. As you inhale, charge yourself with Prana, breathing into the top of your right lung, inflating it. Let go of tension with each exhalation, releasing from the back of your left lung, relaxing it closer to the earth. In this way, you can breathe yourself deeper into the pose.
6. Hold for at least five breaths and then repeat on the other side.

Knees to the Side with Eagle Legs

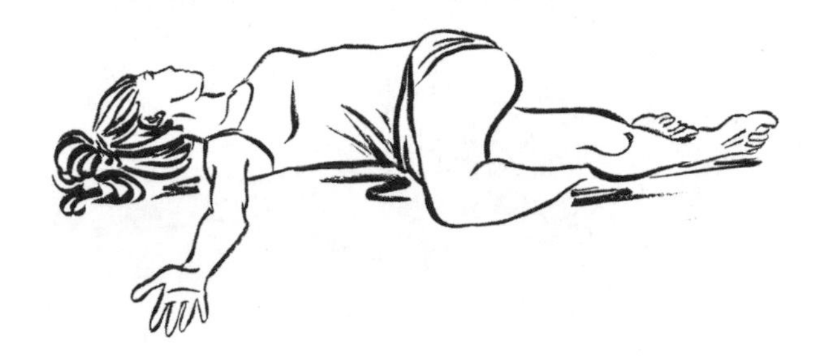

1. Lie on your back, placing your feet on the floor.
2. Cross your left thigh over your right. If you're really flexible, you'll be able to tuck your left toes behind your right leg.
3. Bring your arms out to T position, palms facing up.
4. With your inhalation, delight in your breath fully, drawing your knees into your chest.
5. As you exhale, let go of your worries and drop your legs over to the right. Be sure your left shoulder blade stays grounded.
6. Your back right rib lifts up and over to the left. Use your breath to move deeper into the pose.
7. Hold for at least five breaths and then repeat on the other side.

Knee Down Twist

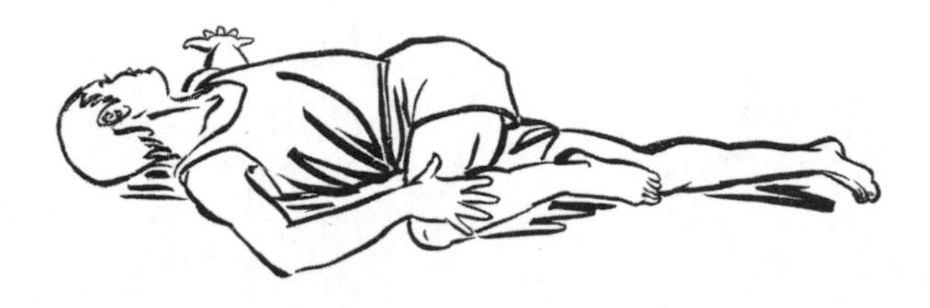

1. Lie on your back with your arms out in T position, palms facing up.
2. Place your right foot on your left thigh. You can rest your left hand on top of your right knee.
3. Receive a deep breath. With your exhalation, drop your right knee over to the left. Keep your left leg steady, flexing your foot.
4. Turn your head to the right, and release your right shoulder into the floor.
5. Inhale into your top left lung. Exhaling, release from the back of your right lung.
6. Hold for at least five breaths and then repeat on the other side.

Twisted Puppy

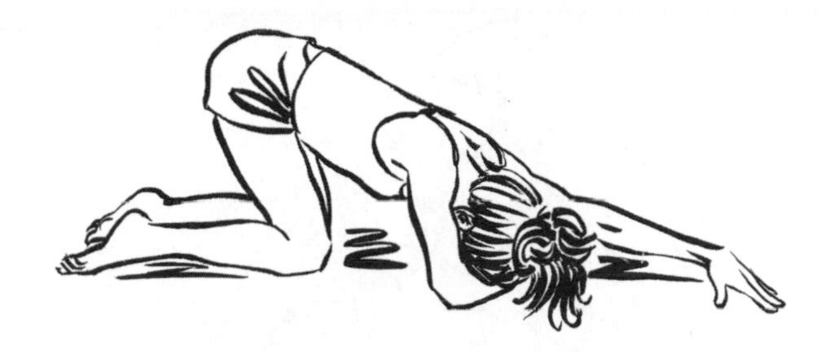

1. Come into Child's Pose.
2. Lift your buttocks up in the air 12 inches higher.
3. Elongate your arms by walking your fingers along the floor away from you.
4. As you inhale, nourish yourself, draw from your fingers into your heart, plugging your shoulders into their sockets. Lift your elbows and armpits as you draw your shoulder blades flat on your back.
5. As you exhale, with gratitude, melt your heart toward the floor. Extend your whole spine, reaching your buttocks back and your arms forward.
6. Walk your hands over to the right, and reach your hips to the left. Breathe into your elongated left ribs.
7. Walk your hands to the left, and reach your hips back to the right, expanding your right side. This is a great back release.

Twisted Downward Facing Dog/ Parivrtta Adho Mukha Svanasana

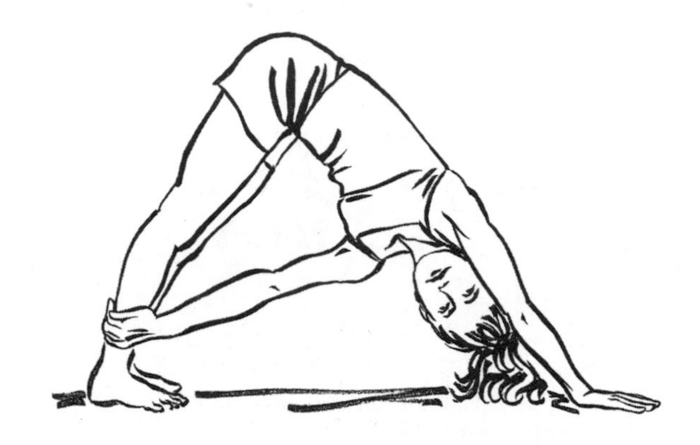

1. Come into Downward Facing Dog. Walk your feet into your hands a few inches.
2. Plug into your desire for absolute freedom, isometrically swiping your hands into each other and drawing from your fingers into your heart.
3. Break free of the chains of self-limitation, pressing the four corners of your hands down into the earth and extending your hips up and back.
4. Keeping your right hand rooted down, lift your left hand and place it on the outer edge of your right leg. (If you can't reach, place your hand on your calf.)
5. Pressing your hand into your leg and your leg into your hand, look under your right armpit, playfully twisting your chest.
6. Keep lifting your hips up and back.
7. Release your hand, and try on the other side.

Simple Seated Twist/ Parivrtta Sukhasana

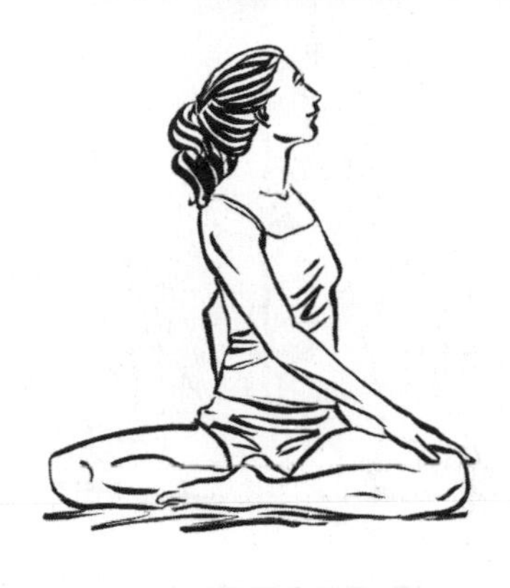

1. Sit in Simple Seated Pose, using a blanket if your lower back needs support or if your hips are tight.
2. Place your right fingertips on the floor (or blanket) directly behind your right hip. Rest your left hand on your outer right knee.
3. Hug your legs in as you receive your inherent fullness. With this inhalation, root your tailbone down and lengthen through your crown.
4. As you exhale, turn to the right and twist, releasing toxins, stale air, and tension.
5. Each time you inhale, draw in your legs and sit up taller.
6. Each time you exhale, move into a deeper twist.
7. After five or so breaths, twist to the other side.

Pose to Lord of the Fishes/ Ardha Matsyendrasana

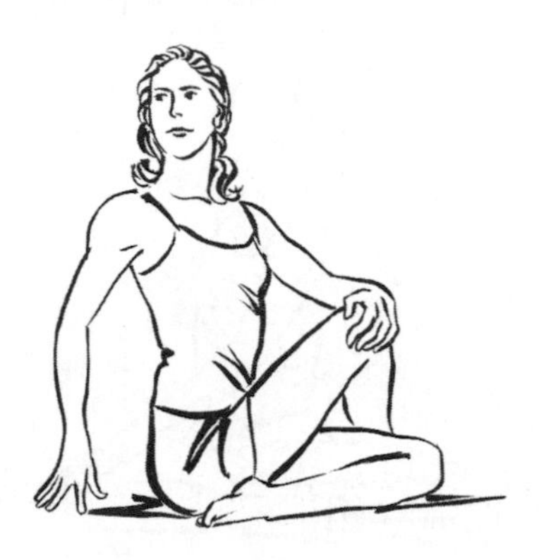

1. Sit in Simple Seated Pose, using a blanket if necessary. Step your right foot to the left of your left thigh. Place your right hand directly behind your right hip to support your back. With your left hand, hold your right knee.
2. As you inhale, hug your legs in and extend your spine in both directions. Your body swells with your true essence.
3. With your exhalation, let go of your limitations, turning and twisting to the right.
4. Breathe into the back of your right lung, expanding it behind you to move from the back of your left ribs more fully into the twist. Be sure your left hip stays steady and does not lift forward.
5. Bend your elbows out slightly, lifting your heart and broadening your chest.
6. Hold for at least five breathes before repeating on opposite side.

Pose to Sage Marichi III/ Marichyasana III

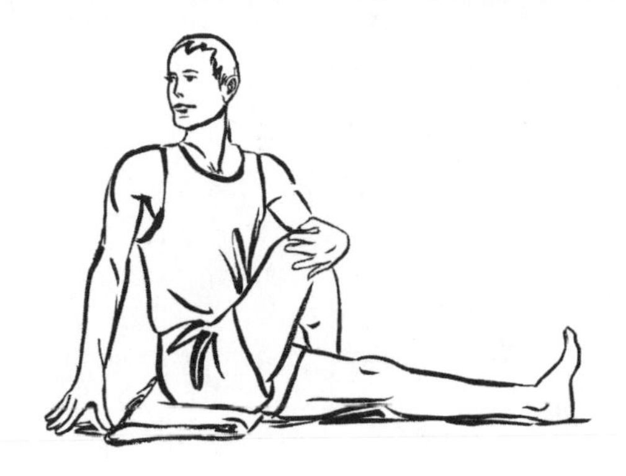

1. Sit on the floor with your legs stretched out in front of you. (If you need to, please sit on a blanket.)
2. Bending your right knee, step your right foot to the left of your left leg. Keep your left foot flexed with your toes pointing up and your leg active.
3. Place your right hand on the floor directly behind your right hip. Rest your left hand on your outer right knee.
4. As you inhale, draw from your feet up into your pelvis and hug your legs in, aligning with your stability. From that strength, allow the freedom of the breath to lift your heart and lengthen your spine.
5. As you exhale, move your left back forward to twist. Expand the back of your right lung behind to deepen.

6. Bend your elbows out so your collarbone and chest expand. Actively lift your heart, offering out your fullness.
7. Hold for at least five breaths before repeating on opposite side.

Pose to Sage Bharadvaja/ Bharadvajasana

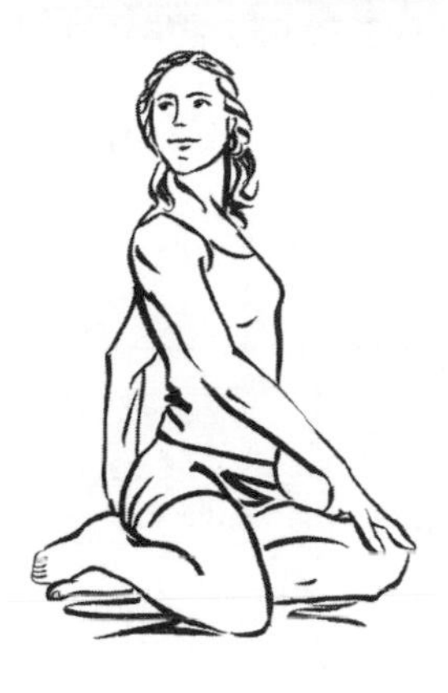

1. From a seated position, swing both legs to the left so both heels are next to your left hip and your knees are pointing to the right. You may need to sit up on a blanket.
2. Use your right hand behind your right hip to support your lower back. Place your left hand on your outer right knee.
3. Open to receive your breath, and feel yourself expanding form the inside out. Let this inner brightness lengthen your spine and lift your heart.
4. Keeping this expansiveness, twist to the right with your next exhalation. Keep your left hip heavy and steady, twisting only from your ribs.
5. Your lower belly and heart lift as your spine lengthens and your ribs soften.

6. Slowly turn your head to the left. As you look over your left shoulder, deepen your twist to the right by initiating from your back-body.
7. Hold for at least five breaths. With your exhalation, turn your head back to neutral and then release the twist. Repeat on the opposite side.

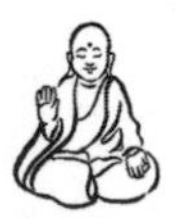

Be Mindful

Remember you need to root in order to rise. Keep your hips, especially your back hip, heavy and you'll have more freedom to twist.

Chapter 11

Moving Within: Seated Forward Bends

Forward bends are internal and introspective. As a turtle crawls into its shell, you also move inside as you fold. Your sense organs get less stimuli, and your nervous system cools and quiets. When you fold forward, you practice humbleness, bowing to all those who have come before you, who have made you who you are today.

Physiologically, forward bends tone the digestive organs, as well as the liver and kidneys. The legs—particularly the hamstrings—the buttocks, and the lower back stretch. Done with proper alignment, forward bends can release the lower back.

Within every seated forward bend is a backbend, as the lower back must gently arch. This results in a lengthening of the spine.

If you have tight hamstrings, forward bends can be quite challenging. Remind yourself that yoga practice is not about performance. Create balance within, and don't worry how deep you go in the pose. To assist your forward bends, sit up on a blanket.

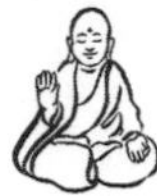

Be Mindful

Most people tend to extremely round their backs while doing seated forward bends. This compression won't release the lower back and may aggravate any existing conditions.

Let's see how alignment applies to seated forward bends:

- The Focal Point for all seated forward bends is the core of the pelvis.
- Inner Spiral is emphasized. The pelvis must tilt forward. Think back bend. The lower spine lifts in and up, making the lower back concave. The heart lifts and expands.
- The spine lengthens in two directions: down through the tailbone and up through the crown.
- The thighs stay rooted. Lifting them tightens the hamstrings and back.
- Think extension rather than bending forward. The torso lengthens. Again, it's not about how deep you go. Can you reach your heart out more fully?

As with the rest of the book, this entire chapter can be used as a sequence. For a great variation, practice the first four poses on one side before doing them on the opposite side.

Some Forwardbend Cautions

If you have back issues, be very mindful that you don't round and collapse your back, as this compresses your spine. Concentrate on Inner Spiral, and try to create as much length in your back as possible.

Please do not lift your thighs to get lower. This may initially feel like a great stretch, but it only results in tightening your muscles. The tighter your hamstrings, the more difficult this is. For some, just coming forward an inch makes for a deep forward bend.

If you're pregnant, practice all forward bends with your legs wide enough apart to accommodate your passenger.

Finally, don't forget to use a blanket if necessary.

Head-to-Knee/Janu Sirsasana—Bending Between Both Legs

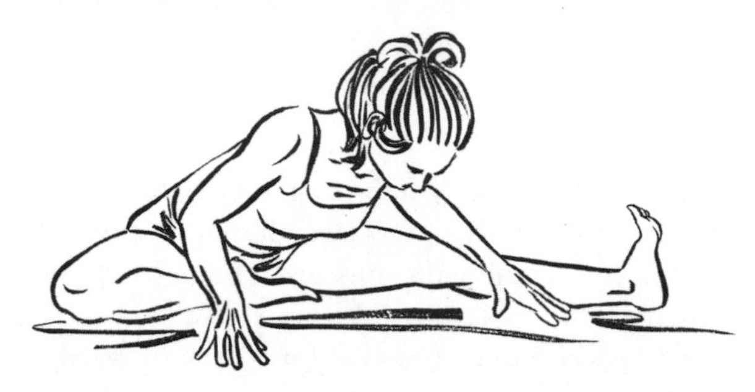

1. Sitting up tall, on a blanket if necessary, extend your right leg out straight in front of you. Bend your left leg. Depending on your flexibility, place your left foot either against the right leg or your heel in your groin.
2. Cup-shape your hands, fingertips touching the floor and palms elevated on the floor between your legs.
3. As you inhale draw, from your right foot and left knee into the core of your pelvis. Turn your thighs slightly in and down, so you're your femurs (thigh bones) root and your pelvis tilts forward. Claw the floor in toward your body; your lower belly and heart lift.
4. As you exhale, offer out your thanks, extending as you bow forward. Let your heart lead the way, imagining someone you love just beyond you. Keep the engagement of your legs as you lengthen from your pelvis out through your feet.

5. Hold for at least five breaths or longer. Repeat with your left leg extended and your right leg bent.

Head to Knee/Janu Sirsasana

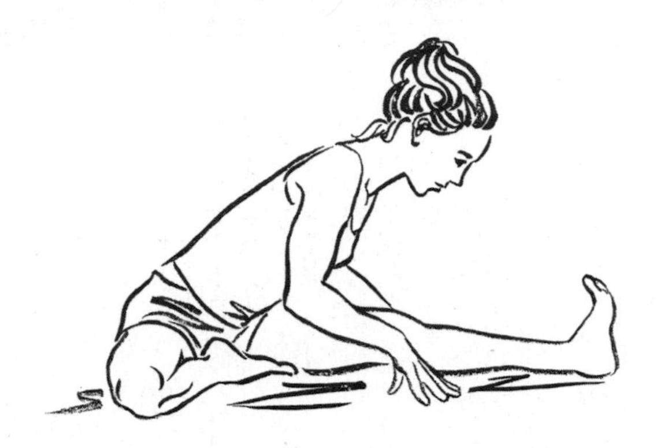

1. Sit with your right leg extended in front of you and your left knee bent. The sole of your left foot should be either against your inner right thigh or your left heel should be back in your groin, making a wider angle between your legs.
2. Cup-shape your hands on the floor on either side of your extended leg.
3. As you inhale, feed the pose, drawing energetically in from your feet and hands into your pelvis.
4. Keeping your legs engaged, gently roll your thighs in toward each other and down toward the floor in Inner Spiral. Your thighs root, and your pelvis tilts forward.
5. As you exhale, bow forward, creating length in your whole spine and legs. Bowing within, keep your whole body expansive and bright as you soften your skin. Soften your senses as you retreat from the outer world.
6. Repeat on the opposite side.

Side Head to Knee/ Parsva Janu Sirsasana

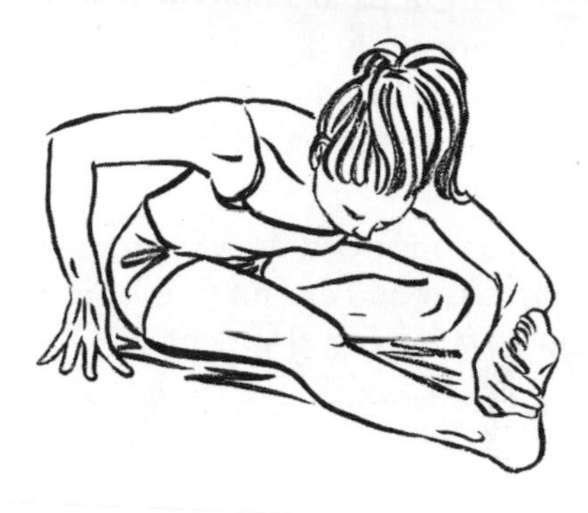

This asana is a spinal twist and forward bend.

1. Sitting with a long spine, extend your right leg out straight in front of you. Place your left foot against your right thigh, or place your heel in your groin.
2. Reach your right hand on the floor (or blanket) behind your right hip, resting your left hand on your right thigh.
3. As you inhale, plug into your strength, drawing your legs energetically in and up into the core of your pelvis.
4. Turn your thighs softly in and down; root your legs while you tilt your pelvis forward. Extend your spine.
5. As you exhale, twist to the right.

6. Walk your left fingers down your outer right leg, leading the pose with your heart first. Be sure your left shoulder blade stays on your back. Move your right hand along the floor by your hip. If you are really flexible and can keep your spine long and shoulder blades flat on your back, try holding onto the right side of your foot with your left hand.
7. To enhance your twist, draw from your right foot into your pelvis and extend from your pelvis out through your left leg. Bow within.

Rotated Head to Knee/ Parivrtta Janu Sirsasana

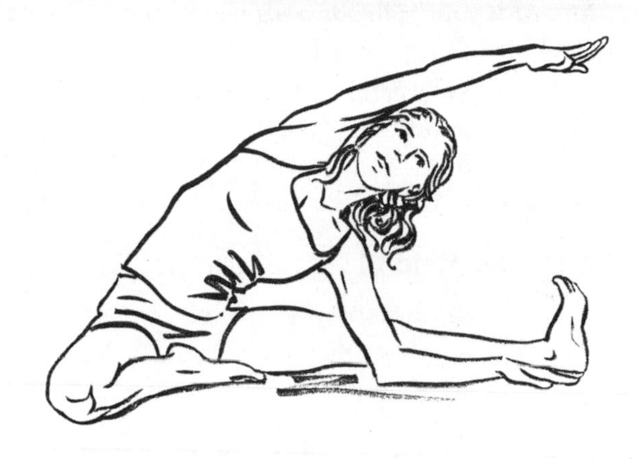

1. Sit in Head to Knee Pose.
2. Place your right hand on the floor in front of your inner right thigh.
3. Inhale your left arm overhead. Draw from your fingers into your heart and your legs into your pelvis, creating a strong container for your energy.
4. As you exhale, extend your torso as you reach your left arm toward your right toes.
5. Walk your right fingers along the floor away from your legs so your right ribs lower and your left ribs stack on top of them. You can either leave your hand here, increasing your twist, or, without losing the twist, slide your hand back along side your leg.

6. Let your heart shine out, and extend your left arm and legs. Keep your left buttock grounded. If you're really flexible, grasp onto your right foot with your right or both hands, keeping your chest open.
7. Hold for five breaths to one minute before doing the opposite side.

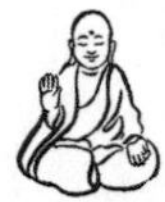

Be Mindful

If you are really flexible, you can grasp onto your big toe with both hands. Root your bottom elbow into the earth and extend your top elbow upward. Open your heart toward the sky.

Wide-Legged Forward Bend/ Upavistha Konasana

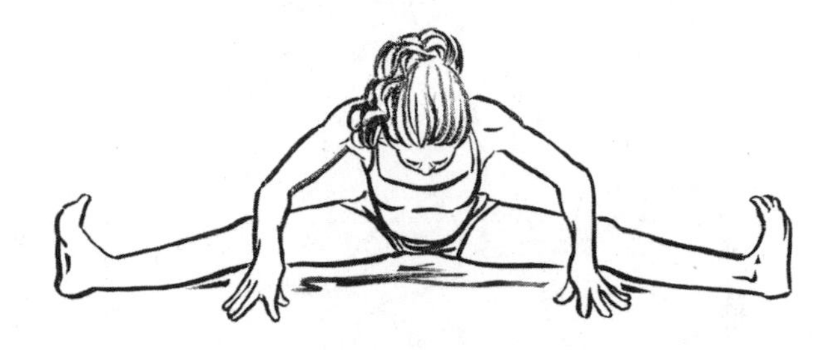

1. Sit with your legs wide apart, up on a blanket if necessary.
2. Manually Inner Spiral your legs, one leg at a time: remove your buttocks cheek away from your sitz bone. With one hand on the top of your thigh and one on the bottom, roll your thigh slightly down as the back of your thigh widens out.
3. With flexed feet, embrace your energy fully. Draw from your heels into your pelvis.
4. Place your fingertips on the floor. As you inhale, claw the floor and roll your inner thighs in and down.
5. Keeping your spine long, as you exhale, bow forward with a full heart in self-honoring.
6. Without losing engagement, reach enthusiastically out from your feet as if you are "stepping" on the wall.

Full Forward Bend/ Paschimottanasana

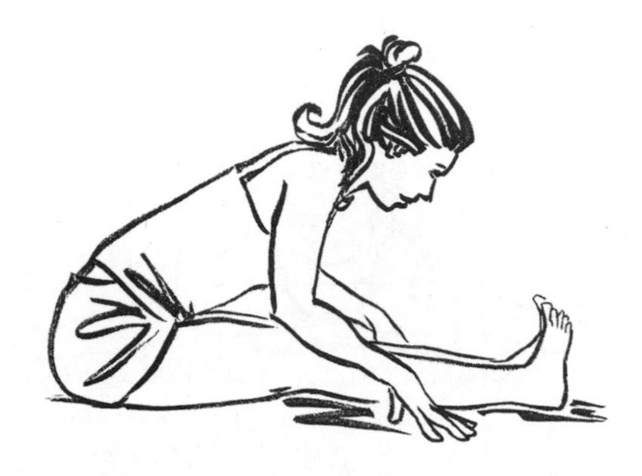

1. Sit with your legs extended out in front of you, your feet flexed.
2. Think Mountain Pose, and engage your legs. Draw from your feet actively into your pelvis, feeding the pose.
3. Inhale, and your heart swells with gratitude as you claw the floor. Subtly move your thighs in toward each other and down, tilting your pelvis forward.
4. With your exhalation, bow forward and reach your heart out, visualizing a person you are grateful for just beyond your toes.
5. If you're really flexible and can keep your back relatively flat and your shoulder blades flat on your back, grasp onto the outer edges of your feet. Otherwise, keep clawing the floor.
6. Hold for at least five deep breaths.

Chapter 12

Receiving: Relaxation and Meditation

In our quick-paced and multitasking society, it's rare to find time to relax. Carving out time for relaxation releases tension from the body and allows your nervous system to calm. Taking this time recharges your batteries, helping you be more alert and productive.

This chapter contains some restorative postures that recharge the body. Restorative asanas were originally intended for people with illness or injuries but later proved to greatly reduce stress. The nervous system is also soothed, and the breath can flow freely. In restorative poses, props support your body so you can release fully. These poses are generally held for a long time—5 minutes and longer. I recommend holding these poses for at least 10 minutes, as that's the time it takes your nervous system to settle. The longer you hold, the greater the benefits.

Relaxation/*Savasana* is the most practiced restorative pose. This pose should always be the final pose of your asana practice, as holding this pose allows your body to "digest" the effects of your practice and provides a time of integration. In Savasana, you lie on your back, maintaining full awareness, experiencing yourself in the moment, receiving your practice, your breath. You develop the art of letting go. Because this restorative pose is the finale of your practice, Savasana should be held for at least 10 minutes for the full benefits of relaxation. This extra time spent assimilating what you've received will revitalize you more for the rest of your day or evening.

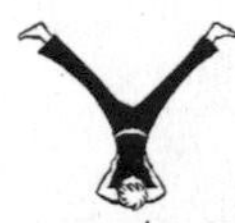

Yoga Speak

Savasana is the most important asana of your practice. It is the relaxation you do at the end of your practice. Savasana literally means "Corpse Pose."

Key Points for Relaxation and Restorative Poses

There are a few things to keep in mind for restoratives, including relaxation:

- Try to keep still. Once you adjust, settle yourself into the pose.
- Focus on your breath. As you inhale, receive nourishment; as you exhale, let go of tension.

- Stay aware of sensation. Do so, mindfully, without judgment. Try your best not to fall asleep.
- Hold the poses for 10 minutes.

It's important to release all these poses gradually. You can lose the benefits of these asanas if you sit up quickly. This jars the nervous system in particular. To release a restorative pose, including Savasana:

1. First deepen your breath.
2. Slowly wake up your body, wiggling your fingers and toes.
3. Roll over to one side in fetal position for a few breaths.
4. Keeping your legs heavy, use your hands to press yourself up.
5. Take at least a few moments to sit and be. (This is a great time for meditation.)

Time for Meditation

Meditation has long been proven to have a positive effect on brain chemistry, helping practitioners relax. Meditation has been found to reduce the effects of stress; for example, lowering high blood pressure and enhancing the immune system. Yoga developed as a practice to condition the body for long hours of meditation, as it's easier to sit when your body has been opened.

Although most of us don't have the time to meditate for several hours a day, you might be able to integrate sitting in meditation for 10 minutes to 1 hour. You'll find benefits in meditating even for a few minutes a day. Try to incorporate meditation into your practice before or after Savasana. The more you practice meditation, the easier it will be to sit for longer periods of time.

Concerns and Cautions

Before you get into the poses in this chapter, please keep a few cautions in mind:

- If you experience lower back pain in Savasana, try Supported Savasana instead.
- If you're pregnant, it's not recommended that you lie on your back after the first trimester. This hinders the flow of oxygen to your baby. Try lying on your side with two pillows under your head so your bottom shoulder doesn't get crushed. Also place a pillow or blanket between your knees.
- For some mental illnesses, Savasana and other types of meditation with closed eyes are not recommended for everyone. If your doctor does not recommend meditation, try Restorative Fish with your eyes open instead.

Restorative Fish/ Restorative Matsyendrasana

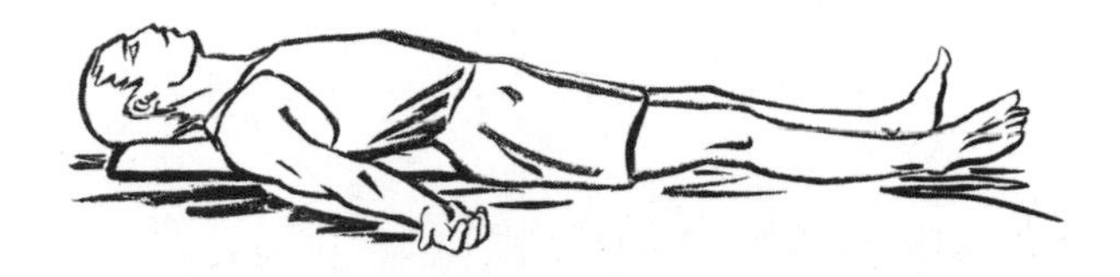

1. Roll up a blanket or your mat. (A sticky mat rolls to the ideal size.) This prop needs to be as long as your spine and about 4 inches thick.
2. Sit on the floor with your legs extended, your buttocks against your blanket, touching it but not sitting on it. Now lie down with your back on your blanket. It should be in line with your spine.
3. Release your arms on either side of you, palms facing up. Bending your elbows slightly to increase your shoulder blades' ability to drop down around the blanket.
4. Close your eyes and receive your breath. Feel your inhalation washing up your body as your whole body expands with nourishment.
5. As you exhale, your breath washes down your body and your whole body softens. Your shoulder blades release around your blanket, and your

heart opens. This pose is great for those with breathing or shoulder difficulties and for releasing anxiety.

6. Release the pose gently.

Corpse Pose/Savasana

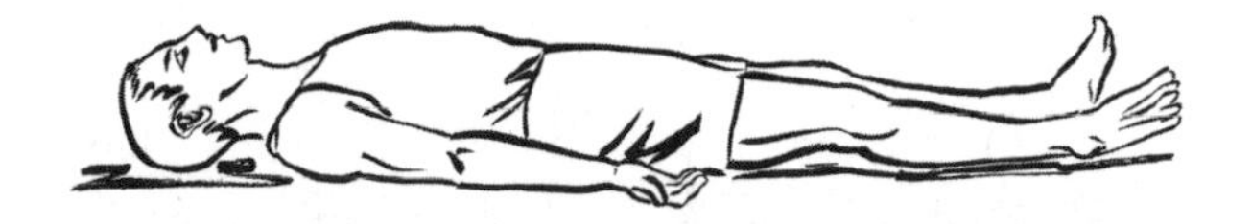

1. Lie flat on your back. Start out in a prone Mountain Pose/Tadasana, with your legs together and your body straight. Your shoulder blades are flat on your back, and your arms out to your sides with your palms facing up.
2. Close your eyes. Focus your awareness on your breath.
3. As you exhale, allow your body to relax and let go. Your feet will probably drop apart. With each inhalation, your body receives. With each exhalation, your body becomes heavier as it releases fully.
4. After settling into your breath, you might want to concentrate on progressively relaxing your whole body, each part at a time. Start by relaxing your feet, and work your way up your body to your head.
5. When you finished this progressive relaxation, soften into your breath and into this moment. This is your time to receive. You have nothing to do and nowhere to go. Just be.
6. Release the pose gently.

Supported Corpse Pose/ Supported Savasana

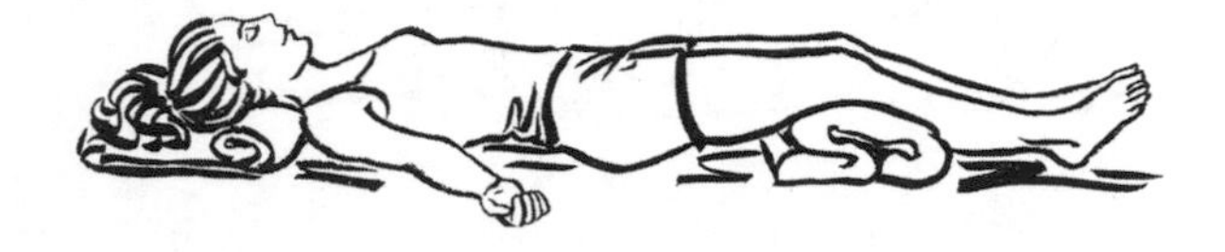

You need two blankets for this pose (or one pillow and a blanket).

1. Sit on the floor with your legs extended out in front of you. Place a rolled blanket or pillow under your knees. (This is ideal if your lower back bothers you when you lie on the floor.)
2. Roll a second blanket thinly to support the curve of your neck, just at the natural arch, so your head rests back and your neck is in line with the rest of your spine. Lie back and adjust your neck support.
3. Close your eyes and open to receive your breath and sensation. With each exhalation, allow your whole body to relax and let go. Let yourself be nourished.
4. Release the pose gently.

Meditation

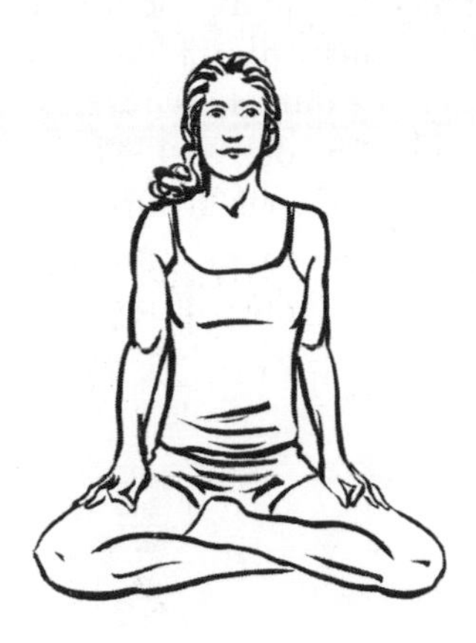

1. Sit in a comfortable seated position. (For some variations on seated poses, see Chapter 2.) If you need support, sit on a blanket, chair, or even with your back against a wall. Sit up tall, with your hands resting on your thighs and close your eyes.
2. As you inhale, open to receive your fullness. Your heart and chest expand as your spine lengthens.
3. Draw the back of your ears behind you until the base of your skull is over your tailbone. Your shoulder blades magnetize to the back of your heart.
4. Keeping your internal brightness, allow your outer body to soften. Your skin releases and your shoulders and ribs soften.
5. Bring your awareness to your breath. Focus on your nostrils where the breath enters and leaves. Allow this sensation and the sound of your

breath to be at the forefront. Move all other sounds, thoughts, and distractions to the background. Your mind will wander. When it does, acknowledge the thought without judgment and then let it go with your next exhalation. Return to the sensation of your breath with your next inhalation. Continue concentrating on your breath for a few minutes or more.

Chapter 13

Taking It with You: Brief Practices

There will be times when you're unable to take a yoga class. Perhaps you're at work, traveling, feeling under the weather, or just too busy. Maybe you want to explore a yoga practice on your own. In this chapter, you find four brief organized practices.

You can make these practices longer by adding various asanas from the other chapters of this book. In fact, the whole book is organized so you can use it as a practice as well. (The chapters are written in the order you should practice.) You could also pick several asanas from each chapter to create a self-tailored practice. It is ideal to add different poses to your practice so you cover different asanas on each day, rather than repeating all the same poses over and over. However, there should be some continuity to your practice. You will notice that some asanas get repeated in each of the practices; these key poses should be repeated.

For the last sequence in this chapter, adapt it to fit your location—you're probably not going to want to sit on the floor in your office. Instead, you can do the seated poses in your office chair. When traveling, try to find a quiet corner of the airport to practice while you're waiting for your flight. Or take a break from driving and do a few poses at a rest area.

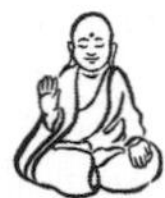

Be Mindful

Please only try the following practices if you have read through the entire book, going over the alignment information and the precautions for each asana category.

Charging Your Battery: Practice for Energy

Time: 1 hour or longer, depending on how long you hold poses and meditate.

1. Seated Pose with Full Yogic Breathing (Chapter 2)
2. Sun Breaths (Chapter 3)
3. Downward Facing Dog into Plank into Downward Facing Dog (Chapter 3)
4. Uttanasana Flow (Chapter 3)
5. Sun Salutation—regular set (each side) (Chapter 3)
6. Sun Salutation with Warrior I instead of Lunge (1 on each side) (Chapters 3 and 4)

7. Sun Salutation with Side Plank (1 on each side) (Chapters 3 and 6)
8. Warrior II into Reverse Warrior II on right side (Chapter 4)
9. Repeat on left side
10. Extended Side Angle into Triangle into Half Moon into Sugar Cane Stick into Triangle (Chapter 4)
11. Repeat on left side
12. Uttanasana (Chapter 4)
13. Standing Split (Chapter 4)
14. Handstand or Handstand Prep (Chapter 6)
15. Extreme Side Stretch into Warrior III on right side (Chapter 4)
16. Repeat on left side
17. Wide-Legged Forward Bend (Chapter 4)
18. Knee Down Lunge (both sides) (Chapter 5)
19. Knee Down Lunge with Quad Stretch (both sides) (Chapter 5)
20. Pigeon Prep and/or Pigeon (both sides) (Chapter 5)
21. Crane Prep and/or Crane (Chapter 6)
22. Half Boat and/or Boat (Chapter 6)
23. Headstand Prep or Headstand and then release into Child's Pose (Chapter 8)
24. Bridge (Chapter 9)
25. Repeat Bridge or Upward Facing Bow (2 or more times) (Chapter 9)

26. Knee Down Twist (Chapter 10)
27. Pose to Lord of the Fishes or Pose to Sage Marichi (Chapter 10)
28. Head-to-Knee series (Chapter 11)
29. Full Forward Bend (Chapter 11)
30. Meditation (Chapter 12)
31. Savasana for 10 minutes (Chapter 12)

Something's Better Than Nothing: Practice When Time Is Limited

1. Seated Pose with Full Yogic Breathing (Chapter 2)
2. Child's Pose into Downward Facing Dog (Chapter 3)
3. Forward Bend (Chapter 3)
4. Sun Salutation (3 times) (Chapter 3)
5. Mountain (Chapter 3)
6. Warrior II (Chapter 4)
7. Extended Side Angle (Chapter 4)
8. Warrior I (Chapter 4)
9. Headstand Prep or Headstand and then release into Child's Pose (Chapters 8 and 3)
10. Knee Down Lunge (Chapter 5)
11. Half Frog (Chapter 5)
12. Half Bow (Chapter 9)
13. Bow (Chapter 9)
14. Twisted Puppy (Chapter 10)

15. Simple Seated Twist (Chapter 10)
16. Head to Knee over Straight Leg (Chapter 11)
17. Full Forward Bend (Chapter 11)
18. Savasana for at least 5 minutes (Chapter 12)
19. Meditation (Chapter 12)

Slow and Steady: Relaxation Sequence for Hectic Days

1. Restorative Fish (Chapter 12)
2. Circling Joints (Chapter 3)
3. Cat and Dog (4 to 10 times) (Chapter 3)
4. Child's Pose (Chapter 3)
5. Sphinx (Chapter 5)
6. Half Pigeon (Chapter 5)
7. Cobra Variation (Chapter 9)
8. Puppy (Chapter 3)
9. Twisted Puppy (Chapter 10)
10. Knee Down Twist (Chapter 10)
11. Big Toe series (Do this lying on your back, and use a strap.) (Chapter 4)
12. Legs Against the Wall (Chapter 9)
13. Knees to Side (Chapter 10)
14. Restorative Savasana for 10 minutes (Chapter 12)

Take a Break: Practice for Work and Travel

1. Seated Pose with Full Yogic Breathing (You can do this in a chair if you need to.) (Chapter 2)
2. Forward Bend Flow (You can do this in a chair.) (Chapter 3)
3. Downward Facing Dog (You can do this standing or with your hands against a wall.) (Chapter 3)
4. Warrior I or Lunge (Chapter 4)
5. Extreme Side Stretch (This pose counterbalances sitting for long periods.) (Chapter 4)
6. Cobra Variation (Do this standing.) (Chapter 9)
7. Simple Seated Twist (Chapter 10)
8. Wide-Legged Forward Bend with Hands Clasped Behind Back (Chapter 4)
9. Meditation (Chapter 12)
10. Savasana (can do seated if necessary) (Chapter 12)

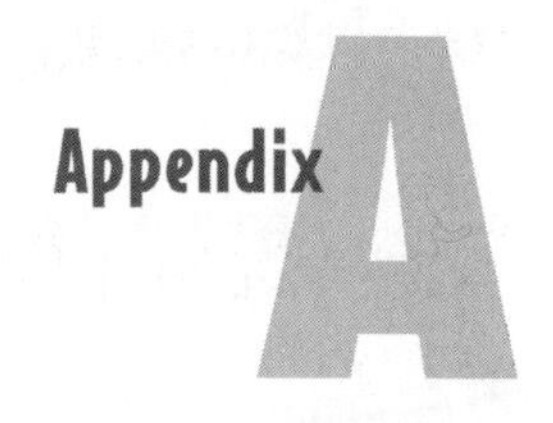

Appendix A

Glossary

agni Literally "fire," agni can refer to heat within the body that increases circulation and secretions.

Anjali Mudra *Anjali* literally means "to extend forth offering." *Mudra* means "seal." In this mudra, the hands are together in a prayer position over the heart.

apana vayu One of the five main Pranas, apana vayu is a downward-flowing energy. It governs the area from the navel down, assisting with elimination, reproduction, and digestion. Try a sighing exhalation and you'll feel the releasing effects of apana vayu on the nervous system.

asana Literally means "seat." Asanas are Hatha Yoga postures.

Astanga Yoga Part of Raja Yoga, Astanga literally means "Eight Limbs."

balanced action Having a balance of energies within an asana. Some examples are a balance between engaging and softening, integration and extension, receiving and giving, discipline and spontaneous play, and taking it to the next level and respecting your limitations.

block A prop used in yoga, a block is a wooden, foam, or cork rectangle about 4×6×9 inches. Blocks are used as extension for the arms to touch the floor or for stability and support.

chakra One of the seven major centers where energy is received, processed, and transmitted. The word literally means "wheel" or "disc."

feet parallel A position in which you line up your second toe (your big toe being toe number one and your pinky toe being toe number five) with the middle of your ankles and middle of your knees.

The Five Principles of Alignment Five steps that govern alignment in any pose within yoga or life. These principles are always done in order and add to the previous steps. The Five Principles are Open to Grace, Muscular Energy, Inner Spiral, Outer Spiral, and Organic Energy.

Focal Point Where energy is directed, collected, and radiated out in an asana. There are three Focal Points; only one is active in each pose.

Four Corners of the Feet The fleshy mound where your foot meets the big toe (big toe mound, not the big toe itself), the inner edge of your heel, the fleshy mound where the foot meets your pinky toe (pinky toe mound), and the outer edge of your heel on each foot. When the Four Corners of each foot are grounded, your arches, kneecaps, and thighs lift and engage.

Four Corners of the Hands The fleshy mound (metacarpal) between your thumb and wrist, where your palm meets your index finger, where your outer wrist meets your hand, and where the base of your pinky finger meets your hand. When these corners are rooted, the arch of the palm lifts.

Hatha Yoga Part of the practice of Royal, or Raja Yoga. Hatha Yoga refers to all physical forms of Yoga. The word *hatha* is a compound word consisting of *ha*, or "sun," and *tha*, or "moon." The word represents the joining of the opposites, the pulsation of life.

hips square When the hips are even in level or height. When posing, keep the hips level rather than moving so deeply that you lose the alignment.

Inner Body The energetic body, which can physically swell, expanding the body from the inside out to contain more Prana. Your outer body drapes over your inner body.

Inner Spiral A tornado-shaped spiral that begins at your feet and expands, widening up your legs into your waist. The action turns your thighs slightly in toward each other and then back and apart so the top of your thighs move back and the back of your pelvis widens behind you. This is the third principle of the Five Principles of Alignment.

isometric exercise When you energetically draw parts of your body in toward each other without moving them and your muscles engage.

melting the heart When your energetic heart softens and expands without losing shoulder alignment or losing your inner expansiveness. Think of an abundant bunch of grapes weighing down a vine. You have much to be thankful for, so your heart swells with gratitude for this abundance.

Muscular Energy When you align with your intention by drawing in, feeling your muscles engaging. Your muscles hug evenly to your bones; you draw from the periphery of your limbs into the core of your body. This is the second principle of the Five Principles of Alignment.

Om The sound of the vibration of the Universe. Often chanted at the beginning and end of class, it is an acknowledgment that we are all part of the interwoven web of life.

Open to Grace The first principle of the Five Principles of Alignment. You open to receive your inherent fullness. It's our attitude that's most fundamental to our practice. Set and intention for your practice and soften into this moment. Inhale and open to receive your breath, feeling your body shine from the inside out. Swell with the fullness of life.

Organic Energy The last principle of the Five Principles of Alignment. Organic Energy is a energetic lengthening from the Focal Point out through the legs, arms, or both ends of the spine and head.

Outer Body The skin softens like a cloth draping over your internally expansive Inner Body. You want to relax and soften your body without losing this extra Prana.

Outer Spiral A spiral that moves opposite of Inner Spiral yet complements it. You keep your inner thighs back as you subtly scoop your tailbone. Outer Spiral tones the buttocks. It is the fourth principle of the Five Principles of Alignment.

Prana Life force energy. *Prana* is also synonymous with *breath*. You receive Prana from things that enhance the flow of your vitality: breath, sunlight, water, food, anything that inspires and feeds your soul and creativity.

Savasana The relaxation pose done at the end of practice. This restorative pose is the most important asana of practice. Savasana literally means "Corpse Pose."

scooping your tailbone Roots the tailbone straight down. Often the tailbone sticks out behind you like a happy dog wagging its tail; however, this indicates an overarching of the back. Draw your tailbone subtly down so it points toward the earth.

Shakti The power and force of the Universe; the energy that flows through all things. Shakti is another name for the Divine.

strap A prop commonly found in yoga, a strap is used to hold arms or legs in place or as an extension of the arms. Cotton yoga straps have a buckle and are 6 to 10 feet long.

synovial fluid A lubricating fluid secreted by the synovial membrane. Both the membrane and the fluid protect the joints.

Vinyasa Flowing form.

Yoga The Sanskrit word for "yoke" or "union." This signifies our union of the Self with our true nature, as well as the union of the individual with the Divine. There are four types of practices or paths of yoga you can take to feel integrated within yourself and connected with the Divine. Jnana Yoga is knowledge yoga, the study of sacred text; Bhakti Yoga is the yoga of devotion; Karma Yoga is the yoga of action; and Raja Yoga or royal yoga contains within it the practice of Hatha Yoga. *See also* Hatha Yoga and Astanga Yoga.

Appendix B

Resources

In the past few years, yoga has become increasingly popular. Due to this rise in interest, an incredible amount of resources on yoga are available.

Finding a Yoga Teacher

Working with a certified and experienced yoga teacher is very important, especially if you're dealing with any injuries, limitations, or pregnancy. Some certification programs are broad and provide in-depth training, while others are quick, weekend workshops. Look for someone who is certified and affiliated with the Yoga Alliance (www.yogaalliance.org). The Alliance is a monitoring organization set up by various schools in a wide variety of lineages to maintain teaching standards. It has two levels of affiliation, Registered Yoga Teacher (250 hours of training) and Professional Yoga Teacher (500 hours of training). For this affiliation, look for RYT after a teacher's name.

Anusara Teacher Certification (www.anusara.com) has extremely high standards. When you study with an Anusara teacher, you know you're working with a well-trained and inspiring teacher who is well versed in alignment and in working therapeutically with injuries. Most of these teachers have many years of teaching experience and are certified in other lineages as well.

Another well-respected certification with in-depth training is Iyengar Yoga (www.bksiyengar.com).

References and Great Books

There are so many great books out there; these are just a few.

Feuerstein, Georg, Ph.D. *The Yoga Tradition: In History, Philosophy and Practice*. Prescott: Hohm Press, 1998.

Friend, John. *Anusara Yoga Master Immersion Manual.* The Woodlands, TX: Anusara Press, 2005.

———. *Anusara Yoga Teacher Training Manual.* Spring, TX: Anusara Press, 1999.